11-91

FOLK MEDICINE

THE ENCYCLOPEDIA OF
H E A L T H

MEDICAL ISSUES

Dale C. Garell, M.D. • General Editor

FOLK MEDICINE

Marc Kusinitz

Introduction by C. Everett Koop, M.D., Sc.D.

former Surgeon General, U. S. Public Health Service

CHELSEA HOUSE PUBLISHERS

New York • Philadelphia

The goal of the ENCYCLOPEDIA OF HEALTH *is to provide general information in the ever-changing areas of physiology, psychology, and related medical issues. The titles in this series are not intended to take the place of the professional advice of a physician or other health care professional.*

ON THE COVER: The anatomy of the ginseng plant

CHELSEA HOUSE PUBLISHERS
EDITOR-IN-CHIEF   Remmel Nunn
MANAGING EDITOR   Karyn Gullen Browne
COPY CHIEF   Mark Rifkin
PICTURE EDITOR   Adrian G. Allen
ART DIRECTOR   Maria Epes
ASSISTANT ART DIRECTOR   Noreen Romano
MANUFACTURING DIRECTOR   Gerald Levine
SYSTEMS MANAGER   Lindsey Ottman
PRODUCTION MANAGER   Joseph Romano
PRODUCTION COORDINATOR   Marie Claire Cebrián

The Encyclopedia of Health
SENIOR EDITOR   Brian Feinberg

Staff for FOLK MEDICINE
ASSOCIATE EDITOR   LaVonne Carlson-Finnerty
SENIOR COPY EDITOR   Laurie Kahn
EDITORIAL ASSISTANT   Tamar Levovitz
PICTURE RESEARCHER   Sandy Jones
DESIGNER   Robert Yaffe

First Printing
1   3   5   7   9   8   6   4   2

Library of Congress Cataloging-in-Publication Data

Kusinitz, Marc.
   Folk medicine/by Marc Kusinitz; introduction by C. Everett Koop.
      p. cm.—(The Encyclopedia of health. Medical issues)
   Includes bibliographical references and index.
   Summary: A look at how folk medicine varies in different cultures and how it affects modern medicine.
   ISBN 0-7910-0083-4
          0-7910-0520-8 (pbk.)
   1. Folk medicine—Juvenile literature. [1. Folk medicine.] I. Title. II. Series.
GR880.K94 1991   91-19627
398'.353—dc20   CIP

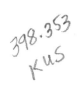
CONTENTS

THE ENCYCLOPEDIA OF
H E A L T H

THE HEALTHY BODY

The Circulatory System
Dental Health
The Digestive System
The Endocrine System
Exercise
Genetics & Heredity
The Human Body: An Overview
Hygiene
The Immune System
Memory & Learning
The Musculoskeletal System
The Nervous System
Nutrition
The Reproductive System
The Respiratory System
The Senses
Sleep
Speech & Hearing
Sports Medicine
Vision
Vitamins & Minerals

THE LIFE CYCLE

Adolescence
Adulthood
Aging
Childhood
Death & Dying
The Family
Friendship & Love
Pregnancy & Birth

MEDICAL ISSUES

Careers in Health Care
Environmental Health
Folk Medicine
Health Care Delivery
Holistic Medicine
Medical Ethics
Medical Fakes & Frauds
Medical Technology
Medicine & the Law
Occupational Health
Public Health

PSYCHOLOGICAL DISORDERS AND THEIR TREATMENT

Anxiety & Phobias
Child Abuse
Compulsive Behavior
Delinquency & Criminal Behavior
Depression
Diagnosing & Treating Mental Illness
Eating Habits & Disorders
Learning Disabilities
Mental Retardation
Personality Disorders
Schizophrenia
Stress Management
Suicide

MEDICAL DISORDERS AND THEIR TREATMENT

AIDS
Allergies
Alzheimer's Disease
Arthritis
Birth Defects
Cancer
The Common Cold
Diabetes
Emergency Medicine
Gynecological Disorders
Headaches
The Hospital
Kidney Disorders
Medical Diagnosis
The Mind-Body Connection
Mononucleosis and Other Infectious Diseases
Nuclear Medicine
Organ Transplants
Pain
Physical Handicaps
Poisons & Toxins
Prescription & OTC Drugs
Sexually Transmitted Diseases
Skin Disorders
Stroke & Heart Disease
Substance Abuse
Tropical Medicine

PREVENTION AND EDUCATION: THE KEYS TO GOOD HEALTH

C. Everett Koop, M.D., Sc.D.
former Surgeon General,
U.S. Public Health Service

The issue of health education has received particular attention in recent years because of the presence of AIDS in the news. But our response to this particular tragedy points up a number of broader issues that doctors, public health officials, educators, and the public face. In particular, it points up the necessity for sound health education for citizens of all ages.

Over the past 25 years this country has been able to bring about dramatic declines in the death rates for heart disease, stroke, accidents, and for people under the age of 45, cancer. Today, Americans generally eat better and take better care of themselves than ever before. Thus, with the help of modern science and technology, they have a better chance of surviving serious—even catastrophic—illnesses. That's the good news.

But, like every phonograph record, there's a flip side, and one with special significance for young adults. According to a report issued in 1979 by Dr. Julius Richmond, my predecessor as Surgeon General, Americans aged 15 to 24 had a higher death rate in 1979 than they did 20 years earlier. The causes: violent death and injury, alcohol and drug abuse, unwanted pregnancies, and sexually transmitted diseases. Adolescents are particularly vulnerable because they are beginning to explore their own sexuality and perhaps to experiment with drugs. The need for educating young people is critical, and the price of neglect is high.

Yet even for the population as a whole, our health is still far from what it could be. Why? A 1974 Canadian government report attributed all death and disease to four broad elements: inadequacies in the health care system, behavioral factors or unhealthy life-styles, environmental hazards, and human biological factors.

To be sure, there are diseases that are still beyond the control of even our advanced medical knowledge and techniques. And despite yearnings that are as old as the human race itself, there is no "fountain of youth" to ward off aging and death. Still, there is a solution to many of the problems that undermine sound health. In a word, that solution is prevention. Prevention, which includes health promotion and education, saves lives, improves the quality of life, and in the long run, saves money.

In the United States, organized public health activities and preventive medicine have a long history. Important milestones in this country or foreign breakthroughs adopted in the United States include the improvement of sanitary procedures and the development of pasteurized milk in the late 19th century and the introduction in the mid-20th century of effective vaccines against polio, measles, German measles, mumps, and other once-rampant diseases. Internationally, organized public health efforts began on a wide-scale basis with the International Sanitary Conference of 1851, to which 12 nations sent representatives. The World Health Organization, founded in 1948, continues these efforts under the aegis of the United Nations, with particular emphasis on combating communicable diseases and the training of health care workers.

Despite these accomplishments, much remains to be done in the field of prevention. For too long, we have had a medical care system that is science- and technology-based, focused, essentially, on illness and mortality. It is now patently obvious that both the social and the economic costs of such a system are becoming insupportable.

Implementing prevention—and its corollaries, health education and promotion—is the job of several groups of people.

First, the medical and scientific professions need to continue basic scientific research, and here we are making considerable progress. But increased concern with prevention will also have a decided impact on how primary care doctors practice medicine. With a shift to health-based rather than morbidity-based medicine, the role of the "new physician" will include a healthy dose of patient education.

Second, practitioners of the social and behavioral sciences—psychologists, economists, city planners—along with lawyers, business leaders, and government officials—must solve the practical and ethical dilemmas confronting us: poverty, crime, civil rights, literacy, education, employment, housing, sanitation, environmental protection, health care delivery systems, and so forth. All of these issues affect public health.

Third is the public at large. We'll consider that very important group in a moment.

Fourth, and the linchpin in this effort, is the public health profession—doctors, epidemiologists, teachers—who must harness the professional expertise of the first two groups and the common sense and cooperation of the third, the public. They must define the problems statistically and qualitatively and then help us set priorities for finding the solutions.

To a very large extent, improving those statistics is the responsibility of every individual. So let's consider more specifically what the role of the individual should be and why health education is so important to that role. First, and most obvious, individuals can protect themselves from illness and injury and thus minimize their need for professional medical care. They can eat nutritious food; get adequate exercise; avoid tobacco, alcohol, and drugs; and take prudent steps to avoid accidents. The proverbial "apple a day keeps the doctor away" is not so far from the truth, after all.

Second, individuals should actively participate in their own medical care. They should schedule regular medical and dental checkups. Should they develop an illness or injury, they should know when to treat themselves and when to seek professional help. To gain the maximum benefit from any medical treatment that they do require, individuals must become partners in that treatment. For instance, they should understand the effects and side effects of medications. I counsel young physicians that there is no such thing as too much information when talking with patients. But the corollary is the patient must know enough about the nuts and bolts of the healing process to understand what the doctor is telling him or her. That is at least partially the patient's responsibility.

Education is equally necessary for us to understand the ethical and public policy issues in health care today. Sometimes individuals will encounter these issues in making decisions about their own treatment or that of family members. Other citizens may encounter them as jurors in medical malpractice cases. But we all become involved, indirectly, when we elect our public officials, from school board members to the president. Should surrogate parenting be legal? To what extent is drug testing desirable, legal, or necessary? Should there be public funding for family planning, hospitals, various types of medical research, and other medical care for the indigent? How should we allocate scant technological resources, such as kidney dialysis and organ transplants? What is the proper role of government in protecting the rights of patients?

What are the broad goals of public health in the United States today? In 1980, the Public Health Service issued a report aptly entitled *Promoting Health—Preventing Disease: Objectives for the Nation*. This report expressed its goals in terms of mortality and in terms of intermediate goals in education and health improvement. It identified 15 major concerns: controlling high blood pressure; improving family planning; improving pregnancy care and infant health; increasing the rate of immunization; controlling sexually transmitted diseases; controlling the presence of toxic agents and radiation in the environment; improving occupational safety and health; preventing accidents; promoting water fluoridation and dental health; controlling infectious diseases; decreasing smoking; decreasing alcohol and drug abuse; improving nutrition; promoting physical fitness and exercise; and controlling stress and violent behavior.

For healthy adolescents and young adults (ages 15 to 24), the specific goal was a 20% reduction in deaths, with a special focus on motor vehicle injuries and alcohol and drug abuse. For adults (ages 25 to 64), the aim was 25% fewer deaths, with a concentration on heart attacks, strokes, and cancers.

Smoking is perhaps the best example of how individual behavior can have a direct impact on health. Today, cigarette smoking is recognized as the single most important preventable cause of death in our society. It is responsible for more cancers and more cancer deaths than any other known agent; is a prime risk factor for heart and blood vessel disease, chronic bronchitis, and emphysema; and is a frequent cause of complications in pregnancies and of babies born prematurely, underweight, or with potentially fatal respiratory and cardiovascular problems.

Since the release of the Surgeon General's first report on smoking in 1964, the proportion of adult smokers has declined substantially, from 43% in 1965 to 30.5% in 1985. Since 1965, 37 million people have quit smoking. Although there is still much work to be done if we are to become a "smoke-free society," it is heartening to note that public health and public education efforts—such as warnings on cigarette packages and bans on broadcast advertising—have already had significant effects.

In 1835, Alexis de Tocqueville, a French visitor to America, wrote, "In America the passion for physical well-being is general." Today, as then, health and fitness are front-page items. But with the greater scientific and technological resources now available to us, we are in a far stronger position to make good health care available to everyone. And with the greater technological threats to us as we approach the 21st century, the need to do so is more urgent than ever before. Comprehensive information about basic biology, preventive medicine, medical and surgical treatments, and related ethical and public policy issues can help you arm yourself with the knowledge you need to be healthy throughout your life.

FOREWORD

Dale C. Garell, M.D.

Advances in our understanding of health and disease during the 20th century have been truly remarkable. Indeed, it could be argued that modern health care is one of the greatest accomplishments in all of human history. In the early 20th century, improvements in sanitation, water treatment, and sewage disposal reduced death rates and increased longevity. Previously untreatable illnesses can now be managed with antibiotics, immunizations, and modern surgical techniques. Discoveries in the fields of immunology, genetic diagnosis, and organ transplantation are revolutionizing the prevention and treatment of disease. Modern medicine is even making inroads against cancer and heart disease, two of the leading causes of death in the United States.

Although there is much to be proud of, medicine continues to face enormous challenges. Science has vanquished diseases such as smallpox and polio, but new killers, most notably AIDS, confront us. Moreover, we now victimize ourselves with what some have called "diseases of choice," or those brought on by drug and alcohol abuse, bad eating habits, and mismanagement of the stresses and strains of contemporary life. The very technology that is doing so much to prolong life has brought with it previously unimaginable ethical dilemmas related to issues of death and dying. The rising cost of health care is a matter of central concern to us all. And violence in the form of automobile accidents, homicide, and suicide remains the major killer of young adults.

In the past, most people were content to leave health care and medical treatment in the hands of professionals. But since the 1960s, the consumer of medical care—that is, the patient—has assumed an increasingly central role in the management of his or her own health. There has also been a new emphasis placed on prevention: People are recognizing that their own actions can help prevent many of the conditions that have caused death and disease in the past. This accounts for the growing commitment to good nutrition and regular exercise, for the increasing number of people who are choosing not to smoke, and for a new moderation in people's drinking habits.

People want to know more about themselves and their own health. They are curious about their body: its anatomy, physiology, and biochemistry. They want to keep up with rapidly evolving medical technologies and procedures. They are willing to educate themselves about common disorders and diseases so that they can be full partners in their own health care.

THE ENCYCLOPEDIA OF HEALTH is designed to provide the basic knowledge that readers will need if they are to take significant responsibility for their own health. It is also meant to serve as a frame of reference for further study and exploration. The encyclopedia is divided into five subsections: The Healthy Body; The Life Cycle; Medical Disorders & Their Treatment; Psychological Disorders & Their Treatment; and Medical Issues. For each topic covered by the encyclopedia, we present the essential facts about the relevant biology; the symptoms, diagnosis, and treatment of common diseases and disorders; and ways in which you can prevent or reduce the severity of health problems when that is possible. The encyclopedia also projects what may lie ahead in the way of future treatment or prevention strategies.

The broad range of topics and issues covered in the encyclopedia reflects that human health encompasses physical, psychological, social, environmental, and spiritual well-being. Just as the mind and the body are inextricably linked, so, too, is the individual an integral part of the wider world that comprises his or her family, society, and environment. To discuss health in its broadest aspect it is necessary to explore the many ways in which it is connected to such fields as law, social science, public policy, economics, and even religion. And so, the encyclopedia is meant to be a bridge between science, medical technology, the world at large, and you. I hope that it will inspire you to pursue in greater depth particular areas of interest and that you will take advantage of the suggestions for further reading and the lists of resources and organizations that can provide additional information.

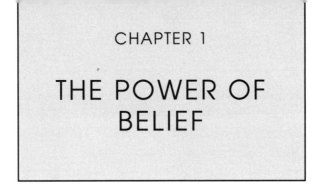

CHAPTER 1

THE POWER OF BELIEF

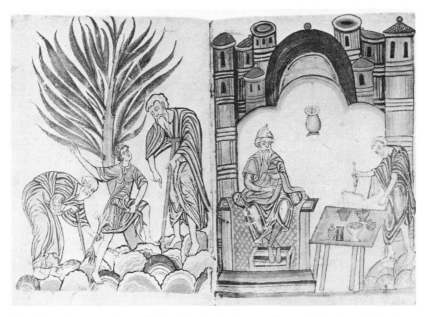

Medieval scene of medicinal herbs being gathered; their use is being determined in a primitive laboratory.

One day in 1973, Max Beauvoir, a scientist trained at both Cornell University and the Sorbonne in Paris, hovered over the bed of his grandfather—one of Haiti's many Voodoo priests—as the old man lay dying.

Often considered to be among the most influential people in a Haitian community, Voodoo priests usually serve as healers, sooth-sayers, exorcists, and counselors. They are an integral part of the country's heritage and social system. So when the grandfather told his university-trained grandson, "You will carry on the tradition," the young man felt he had no choice, according to an account published in the December 15, 1983, *New York Times*. Yet following the old priest's instructions would not be an easy task.

To become a Voodoo priest, Beauvoir's arduous training involved studying all 402 Voodoo spirits as well as the elaborate rites of Voodoo, which were written in the African languages of *Fon* and *Yoruba*. Beauvoir also had to endure secret Voodoo initiation ceremonies, the last of which required him to undergo 41 days of solitary confinement.

FOLK MEDICINE THRIVES

Many people accustomed only to "modern medicine" as practiced in the United States and other Western nations might wonder at Beauvoir's decision to turn toward traditional, or *folk*, medicine. But even some American physicians have learned to respect the powers of ancient healing systems practiced by "uneducated" religious and lay practitioners. For example, in 1987, a weekend course in *ayurvedic medicine*—an important traditional healing art in India—attracted 50 American physicians to the Maharishi Ayurvedic Health Center in Lancaster, Massachusetts. Moreover, in a book published the following

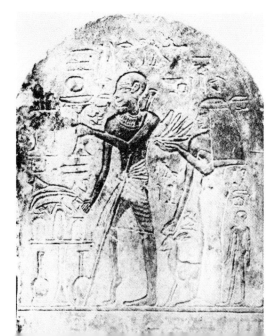

This Egyptian carving, from about 3000 B.C., is the oldest-known record of a female doctor. Here the physician presents her patient, a boy suffering from poliomyelitis, to the goddess Isis to be cured.

year, a psychiatrist, Dr. Carl A. Hammerschlag, described how he combines modern psychiatry with traditional American Indian healing techniques.

Shamans, Voodoo priests, *medicine men*, and other healers who use methods that differ from those used in formal medical science have a history that goes back thousands of years. Despite the incredible advances achieved in medical technology in the 20th century—from antibiotics to heart transplants—these alternative practitioners of the "curing arts" still thrive, finding followers among both the "simple folk" and sophisticated city dwellers around the world.

This does not mean that folk medicine is always effective. A supposed remedy may gain its reputation because it was used to "cure" an ailment that in reality disappeared on its own. Or, in the case of poisoning—such as through a snakebite—the patient's ability to withstand the poison might have been due not to a folk remedy but rather to the fact that some people simply do not become ill from a normally toxic substance. Therefore, it is important to keep in mind that there is a mix of truth and fiction in folk healing traditions.

FOLK HEALERS

Since most people face the threat of disease at some time in their life, every society depends upon certain people to have the knowledge and experience to diagnose and cure sickness. Despite the common goals shared by those who practice folk medicine around the world, however, individual healers and their specific techniques vary greatly among different societies.

Among the Ashanti people of the African country of Ghana, for example, a person with an illness might visit an *herbalist* at his or her home. These healers, who are the general practitioners of that culture, use plants to prepare custom-made remedies for their patients. In the bone-chilling tundras of Siberia, however, the healer, or shaman, is more likely to fall into a trance in order to commune with the supernatural world on behalf of a patient.

Sometimes folk medicine is practiced with rattles and dolls, sometimes with chants, and sometimes with herbs. (Although an herb is,

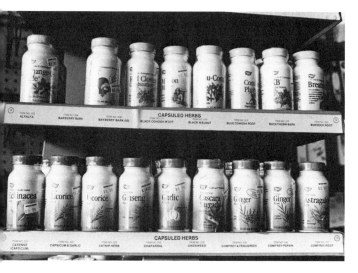

Traditional medicine plays an essential role in world health. Even today, more than 4 billion people seek relief through herbal-based folk treatments.

technically, a specific type of plant, the term is used more loosely when applied to plants used in folk remedies.) Sometimes traditional medicine is practiced by members of the patient's own family, who mix concoctions using recipes that have been handed down through countless generations. Indeed, even when a patient visits a physician schooled in modern medical techniques, he or she will sometimes also visit a folk healer as well.

THE HEALING POWER OF PLANTS

The importance of plants as healing agents is hard to exaggerate: The World Health Organization has estimated that 80% of the world's population rely mainly on traditional medicines for primary health care; a large share of these medications presumably contain plant-based ingredients. For centuries people have amassed empirical knowledge (i.e., knowledge gained through experience and observation) on *herbalism*, the use of plants for healing.

The strong link between plants and healing was demonstrated again quite recently. The *Pacific yew*, a tree found in the forests of the Pacific Northwest, was discovered a few decades ago to contain a chemical known as *taxol*. In the late 1980s, a study from the Johns Hopkins

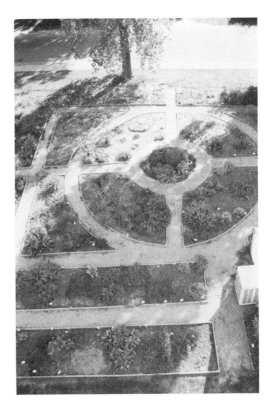

The Medicinal Garden at the University of Rhode Island College of Pharmacy; the garden contains plants possessing important active ingredients, including the Madagascar periwinkle, source of a successful leukemia medication, and foxglove, which can be used to produce the heart drug digitalis.

University School of Medicine showed that the drug was a powerful weapon against ovarian cancer. Later research also indicated that it was very effective against breast cancer and possibly lung cancer as well.

Unfortunately, taxol has been available only in very limited supplies, because it takes six 100-year-old yew trees to produce enough of the drug to treat one ovarian cancer patient, according to an article in the *New York Times* (May 13, 1991). In addition, environmentalists worry that the demand for the cancer drug could prove devastating to the yew population. To avoid such a scenario, scientists have been attempting to find a way to synthesize the taxol molecule so that it can be produced in the laboratory.

THE MEANING OF FOLK MEDICINE

Clearly, traditional medicine is much more than witch doctors, warts, and evil eyes. Throughout the world, much of folk medicine is based on common sense, primitive scientific thinking, and experimentation with cures. Moreover, its importance extends far beyond whether a specific plant will or will not cure a patient's condition. Instead, traditional healing is a mixture of ideas, fears, observations, and faiths that are deeply rooted in the society from which they come. As a result, the healing practices of a people both reflect and influence that group's unique way of looking at the world. It is this set of specific beliefs and practices, developed to cure diseases and maintain health and employed by laypersons, that has come to be known as folk medicine.

The strong influence that this type of medicine maintains throughout the world, then, goes beyond the question of whether a plant truly can or cannot cure a specific illness. It is also very much related to the fact that folk doctors look at the world in much the same way that their patients do, a factor that can be of great importance to an ailing individual seeking the care and skills of a trustworthy healer. It is the faith a patient places in a folk doctor, therefore, and the wise healer's insight into the strong link between the patient's health and his or her

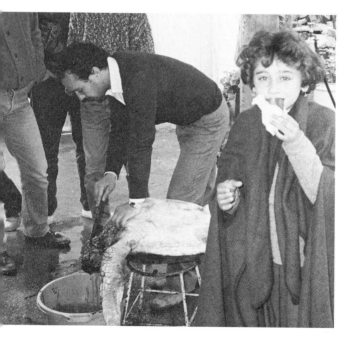

In Beirut, the blood of a sea turtle is consumed by a young girl as a folk remedy for bronchitis.

mental state, that often provide centuries-old treatments with much of their power.

In addition, the knowledge of a society's beliefs and practices with regard to healing is an important tool in building an accurate picture of that society as a whole. This information is also important to health care workers attempting to establish modern, Western-style medical programs in underdeveloped countries. Without such knowledge, these planners would virtually be speaking a foreign language to the local people.

A WARNING

Although folk medicine might seem like little more than a benign practice to many, there are real dangers associated with its use. The federal Centers for Disease Control in Atlanta, Georgia, believes that many herbal medicines imported into this country contain dangerous ingredients.

For example, the drug *chuifong tokuwan,* sold as a painkiller in Texas, was found to contain various prescription drugs as well as the potentially harmful elements lead and cadmium. The U.S. Food and Drug Administration (FDA), which is the major government agency responsible for ensuring that medicines and foods consumed in the United States are safe, issued an alert to its field offices in 1978 warning that chuifong tokuwan must not be allowed across U.S. borders. However, the drug was still being smuggled into the United States from Hong Kong through at least the late 1980s. Other imported folk remedies have contained such ingredients as anabolic steroids (drugs that are often used illegally by athletes to build muscle mass), antibiotics, and even narcotics.

Thus, anyone using folk remedies, including herbal teas, must be aware of the ingredients in the concoctions they consume. By law, legitimate drugs must be manufactured according to strict guidelines, although the consumer often cannot be sure that the substances sold or offered as folk remedies contain only helpful ingredients or at least do not possess any harmful ones.

It is also important to keep in mind that this book is designed to give an overview of the theory and practice of folk medicine, not to instruct readers in the production of herbal remedies for their own use. Although many plants are beneficial to health, others can be deadly. It takes someone skilled in the subject of herbal medicine to know which species can cure and which can kill, how to recognize them when gathering plants in the wild, and how to prepare herbal remedies in a safe and proper manner.

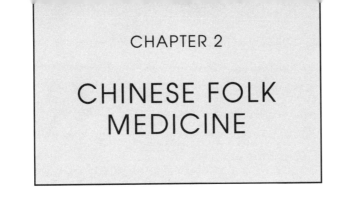

CHAPTER 2

CHINESE FOLK MEDICINE

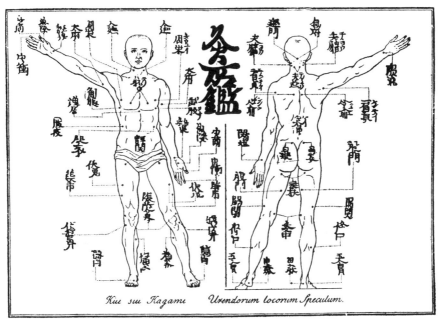

Anatomical diagram of the body's acupuncture points; by inserting needles into the skin, acupuncturists attempt to relieve pain and treat a wide variety of ills.

Although when compared to Western science traditional Chinese healing might be thought of as folk medicine, it is actually much more than a quaint system of old superstitions and family remedies. Rather, this form of health care is steeped in ancient philosophy and practices, relying heavily on notions of the universe as a basis for medical beliefs and stressing harmony and symmetry between the universe and human health.

For example, the number 365 is linked both to the number of days in a year and to the supposed 365 points on the surface of the body where painkilling *acupuncture needles* (discussed later in the chapter) can be inserted.

However, this ancient preoccupation with the idea of symmetry between cosmic forces and the human body apparently long discouraged the scientific study of human anatomy and physiology in China. Well into the 20th century, in fact, battles raged in that nation between those who wanted to bring Chinese medicine into line with the modern concepts of Western health care and those who sought to preserve the deeply rooted philosophies of the ancient healers. Even today, although Western medical concepts are commonly accepted in China, modern health care workers there often work side by side with folk healers.

HEALTH AND HARMONY

If the Chinese medical system could be summed up in just one word, that word might well be *harmony*. To the Chinese, health is a reflection of the natural state of the universe. Good health is thought to depend upon the body's ability to mirror the harmony between heaven and earth. Linked to this concept of health and harmony are three other ideas derived from Chinese philosophy and religion: *Tao, qi,* and *yin/yang*.

Tao

In Chinese philosophy, Tao (the "road" or "way") is the eternal, creative reality that is the source and end of all things; thus, the word signifies "the correct way," or "Heaven's Way." Taoists advocate living in accord with nature, an existence that is both spontaneous and serene.

The philosophy of Taoism had become an organized religion by the 2nd century A.D. Taoist beliefs contributed to the *Great Pharmacopeia*, the 16th-century compendium of treatments based on experiments with minerals, plants, and animal substances. (The book has since been frequently revised and reprinted.)

Qi

More fundamental to Chinese medicine than the *Great Pharmacopeia*, however, is the concept of qi, which means "breaths." According to this idea, as pointed out in the modern text *Survey of Traditional Chinese Medicine*, "The entire universe is nothing but breaths. All that exists either exhales or is itself exhaled, traveling at random and at leisure through time and space." Qi is the force that presides over changes in the human body.

Yin/Yang

As the state of the body changes, so does the balance of two essences within the body that represent the nature of this change. Those essences, yin and yang, have opposite natures and are forever locked in competition. This concept of opposites, always shifting balance in an everchanging universe, is embodied in the concept of yin/yang. Yin and yang are the two forces whose continuous interaction underlies all natural phenomena in the universe, including the functioning of the human body.

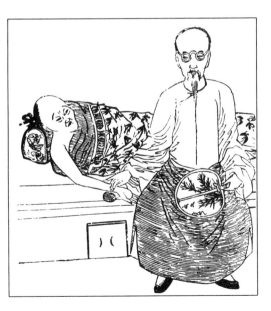

Chinese folk doctors believe that by examining the pulse, a competent physician can not only identify circulatory problems but can determine the state of other internal organs as well.

The ancient texts describe yin as feminine, passive, and negative, as opposed to yang, which is masculine, active, and positive. Yin is hard, whereas yang is soft. Yin represents the moon, earth, water, dampness, darkness, death, evil, ugliness, confusion, and poverty; yang represents heaven, the sun, fire, dryness, light, life, nobility, virtue, beauty, joy, and wealth. In other words, yin and yang represent the two sides to everything. Although yin and yang are always in competition with each other, it is a "cordial competition." Disease is essentially the result of impairment of the proper balance of yin/yang, which, in turn, causes obstruction of the flow of qi throughout the body.

The Art of Taking the Pulse

Because it is believed that yin/yang controls the blood vessels and pulse, the most important part of the healer's diagnosis is considered to be the examination of the pulse, a procedure that can take as long as an hour or more. The *Mai Ching* (Book of the Pulse), written in the 3rd century A.D., is one of the basic works on the traditional Chinese art of pulse taking, a tradition that stretches back 2,500 years.

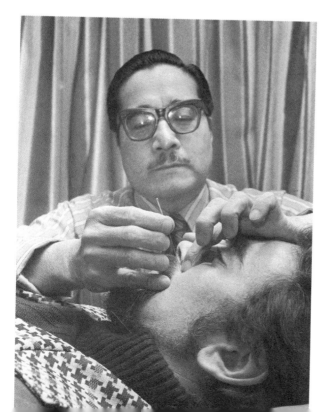

Acupuncture may relieve discomfort by activating the body's own system of natural, painkilling opiates, the endorphins.

Chinese doctors routinely feel not only the radial (wrist) artery, as is commonly done by Western physicians, but also the arteries in the neck and leg. According to Chinese medicine, by merely feeling the pulse a competent doctor should be able to determine the condition of the heart and the aortic valves (which regulate blood flow out of the heart and into the large artery bringing blood to the body), as well as the condition of internal organs.

For example, by exerting slight pressure with the point of the index finger on the left wrist artery, the physician attempts to determine the condition of the small intestine. The doctor applies strong pressure with the point of the middle finger on the right wrist artery in order to analyze the spleen. Thus, according to this system of medicine, by exerting slight or heavy pressure on various arteries with the point of either the index, middle, or third finger, the physician can carry out a comprehensive examination of the patient's internal organs. (In Western medicine, the pulse is used much less extensively; physicians examine it mainly to diagnose heart and circulatory problems.)

TRADITIONAL TREATMENTS

Acupuncture

Several thousand years ago, in order to restore the balance of yin/yang, the Chinese developed acupuncture. This form of treatment consists of inserting needles into any of hundreds of points on the body that are believed to be related in some way to various organs. The technique is used to help relieve problems as varied as neuromuscular pain, arthritis, high blood pressure, gastrointestinal difficulties, and gynecological problems. After the acupuncturist inserts the needles, he or she may twist them or connect them to the source of a small electric current. In China, acupuncturists often supplement the treatment by prescribing medications of plant, animal, or mineral extracts.

Whatever the limits of acupuncture in actually curing disease, the treatment does appear to be effective in relieving pain and is routinely

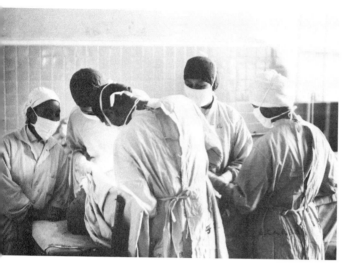

Acupuncture was used as an anesthetic during this thyroid operation in a hospital outside Shanghai.

used in China as an anesthetic during surgery. Many fully conscious patients have undergone complicated operations while being anesthetized through acupuncture only.

One theory about the anesthetic ability of acupuncture is that the insertion of needles activates the body's own system of natural pain-killing opiate chemicals, called *endorphins*. Others have suggested that needle insertion opens certain nerve pathways to the brain, while effectively shutting down the pain nerve pathways from other parts of the body (those undergoing surgery).

Massage: The Healing Hand

Even older than the technique of acupuncture is the instinct to place a hand over a part of the body that is struck, stung, or seized by a cramp and rub the injured area until the pain eases. The ancient Chinese turned this instinct into a highly structured system of massage for reestablishing the balance of yin/yang.

Massage moves the fatty tissue and muscle under the skin and mechanically stimulates the nerve tips. The massage therapist uses his or her fingers and hands to manipulate the body in a variety of ways: thrusting fingers against the skin vertically, in either a circular or back-and-forth motion; grasping the skin and shaking, pressing, rubbing, and pinching; and tapping the skin with the palm, side, or back of the hand or with the fist. Easy massage has an invigorating effect, but vigorous massage has a sedating one, which means that patients with ulcers or other stress-related problems, for example, might be treated with the latter technique.

Massage therapy for children requires modification of classic techniques: Tapping is forbidden and thrusting with fingertips is not considered suitable for children under six years of age.

T'ai chi

The idea that slow, coordinated body motions could help fend off disease or complement other forms of therapy is probably about 1,000 years old. These movements, referred to as *T'ai chi*, are commonly practiced by Chinese adults during morning or evening exercise rituals performed in public.

As in other Chinese therapies, the goal in T'ai chi is to balance yin/yang, in this case by harmoniously linking the mind, sense organs, and internal organs together with the limbs through a series of slow and easy movements.

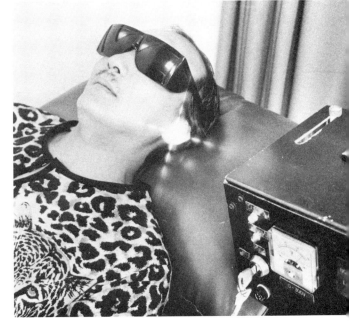

In this high-tech version of acupuncture, laser beams are being used instead of needles to try to cure this patient's smoking habit.

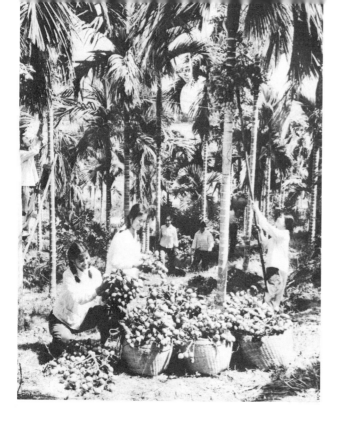

Betel nuts, used as a traditional Chinese medicine, being gathered on China's Hainan Island.

This type of therapy, which at times can look like slow-motion karate, is achieved by concentration, with every movement starting from the sacral area (the section of the backbone forming part of the pelvis and lying between the hips). Motions are carried out in a smooth, uninterrupted, circular direction, with arms and legs moving alternately while the person breathes slowly and deeply.

T'ai chi is thought by practitioners to regulate circulation of the blood and to strengthen joints and ligaments. It is also sometimes practiced to treat high blood pressure, digestive disorders, and the bacterial lung disease tuberculosis.

Herbal Medicine

China's use of plant-based medicines represents thousands of years of experience with the healing properties of hundreds of plants. Over time, treatments have been developed for a variety of ills, including asthma and tuberculosis and disorders of the circulatory system, urinary tract, and gastrointestinal tract.

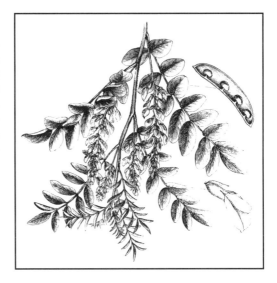

Licorice plant Glycyrrhiza glabra; *the root is used extensively in Chinese folk medicine to treat sore throat, cough, heart palpitations, stomachache, sores, and ulcers.*

Licorice is probably the most extensively used plant in Chinese medicine, and it is frequently added to other prescriptions either to make them more effective or to reduce their toxic effects. Licorice is actually the name commonly applied to 12 different species of plants found in the pea family and belonging to the genus *Glycyrrhiza*. However, it is the root of the plant *G. glabra* that is used so often in folk medicine. The root, which can be mixed into a solution or taken as a powder or pill, is often used to treat sore throat, cough, palpitations (pounding of the heart), stomachache, ulcers, and sores.

The Chinese herb most familiar to Westerners, however, is *ginseng*. Two species of the plant, *Oriental ginseng* (*Panax schinseng*) and *North American ginseng* (*Panax quinquefolium*), are both used in Chinese folk medicine, but in different ways. Oriental ginseng root is often used in combination with other herbs that are themselves used to treat specific conditions. Its role, therefore, is to strengthen the body and help other herbs do their work. On the other hand, North American ginseng root—which has traditionally been popular with southern Chinese (especially the Cantonese)—is often used by these people to cool themselves in summer, to reduce fever, and to relieve fatigue. (The latter species was originally imported to Guangdong Province from the United States.)

Another popular Chinese medicinal herb, *mahuang*, contains *ephedrine*, a drug that stimulates the heart, increases blood pressure, and relaxes bronchial muscles (muscles in the *bronchi*, large passageways leading into the lungs). Ephedrine was used for at least 2,000 years in China before being introduced into Western medicine in 1924, where it proved to be an effective treatment for asthma and other respiratory problems.

Among the hundreds of other Chinese herbal home remedies are bean curd cake for treating the common cold; stewed, unpeeled bananas for hemorrhoids; chrysanthemum flower tea for headaches and bloodshot eyes; dandelion tea for mumps; garlic paste for nosebleed; and an extract of garlic, called *allicin*, to treat bacterial and fungal infections.

BAREFOOT DOCTORS

During the early 1960s, Western health care was making inroads in China as some Chinese officials began encouraging the development of major medical centers and research institutes. But the dramatic and

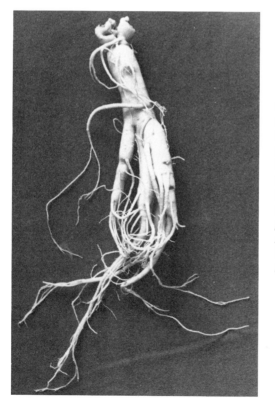

Ginseng root serves a number of purposes in traditional Chinese medicine. Healers use it to help strengthen the body during treatment with other herbs, and a species imported from North America is employed to reduce fever and relieve fatigue.

oftentimes violent Cultural Revolution sparked by the Chinese leader Mao Zedong in 1966, a movement marked by strong anti-Western sentiments, handicapped this effort and forced medical resources to be stretched as broadly as possible. In place of a scarce amount of highly trained physicians, an army of *barefoot doctors* spread out among the enormous population of China.

Barefoot doctors tend to have little or no formal medical education. Instead, they travel throughout the often backward rural areas of the country using acupuncture and herbal remedies to treat common disorders such as colds, influenza, certain skin diseases, and various aches and pains. In this way, medical care reaches even distant parts of China, instead of being concentrated only in areas where more sophisticated treatment is available. Western-style medicine is practiced in cities, of course, but the corps of barefoot doctors and the medicine they practice is just as important to basic health care in this highly populated, economically underdeveloped nation.

CHINESE MEDICINE IN THE UNITED STATES

Although much of Chinese medicine is based on Taoist philosophy— which lacks the "hard" science background of Western medicine—centuries of trial and error have demonstrated that plants do indeed have healing properties, which have been observed and used by Western scientists.

For example, a physician at the UCLA School of Medicine has advised patients with chronic bronchitis (inflammation of the bronchi) to eat spicy foods, such as hot peppers, to break up phlegm and open up air passages.

Moreover, the scientific basis for the healing power of the *ginkgo plant*, a "living fossil" whose ancestors flourished during the time of the dinosaurs, was dramatically demonstrated in 1988, when researchers at Harvard University isolated its *active* component (the chemical responsible for its healing powers), *ginkgolide B*. For thousands of years, a ginkgo leaf extract has been used in Chinese medicine to treat coughs, asthma, acute allergic inflammations, and illnesses of the heart and lungs. Modern British researchers have found

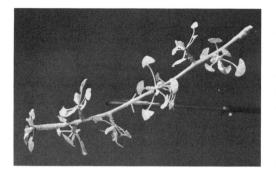

The ginkgo plant, used in Chinese folk medicine for thousands of years, contains a substance known as ginkgolide B. Modern researchers have found this chemical useful in treating asthma and allergic inflammations.

that ginkgolide B is indeed effective in treating people with asthma and allergic inflammations; animal studies by others suggest that it may also be useful in regulating blood pressure and treating kidney disorders.

The *lwallichii* plant provides another example of an ancient remedy that has found a modern use. In 1989, an American researcher received a patent for a synthetic copy of the active ingredient in lwallichii. The ingredient is used to prevent blindness caused by degeneration of the optic nerve and retina. In Japan and China, the plant has long been used to increase blood flow through constricted blood vessels, and this effect appears to contribute to the plant's ability to fight blindness.

Despite the benefits of some medicinal plants, however, a growing Asian population in the United States, coupled with increased importation of Chinese goods, is contributing to the promotion and distribution of useless—and even dangerous—products. Therefore, an unwary consumer of traditional Chinese medications may face potential hazards.

For example, in 1988, California's state health director warned that many Asian medications sold in San Francisco's Chinatown carry inaccurate labeling or contain toxic ingredients. Enouraged by the Oriental Herbal Association and the Chinese Business Herb Association, health officials began distributing a leaflet that lists unproven and dangerous drugs. One product, *cinnabar* sedative pills, may contain mercury and as a result cause serious liver and kidney damage—and ultimately may prove fatal.

Thus, although much Chinese medicine has proved to be of at least some benefit, reckless use of certain products available on the open market can be dangerous.

CHAPTER 3

FOLK MEDICINE OF INDIA

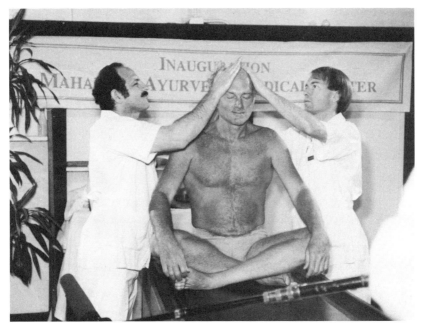

Mike Love, lead singer of the Beach Boys, undergoes oil massage therapy, a technique used in the Indian medical system known as Ayurveda.

According to an ancient legend dating back at least 3,000 years in India, a teacher of folk medicine told his student to search an 8-square-mile area around the teacher's home and to collect all the plants that had no medicinal value. After searching for many hours, the student came back and reported that he could not find a single plant that did not have some medicinal value. This answer pleased the teacher, who then told his student that he was now prepared to enter the healing profession.

It is no surprise that a tale like this would be passed down for so many centuries in India. Healers in that country use hundreds of plant species in more than 8,000 different prescriptions to treat a wide variety of diseases. These folk doctors, in fact, may lead the world in their knowledge of medicinal herbs.

AYURVEDA

Thousands of years ago, such knowledge was recorded and incorporated into a health care system called *Ayurveda* (from *ayuh*, meaning "life," and *veda*, meaning "to know"). Ayurvedic medicine is widely practiced not only in India but in other parts of southern Asia as well, including Pakistan, Nepal, Sri Lanka, and Bangladesh.

The origins of ayurvedic medicine have been somewhat obscured in the mists of time, but it is known that this science is related to the

Ayurvedic healers consider examination of the pulse to be an important part of diagnosis. This ayurvedic doctor, B. D. Triguna, is considered a leading expert on the pulse.

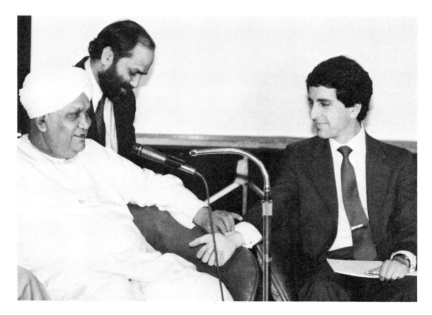

Atharva-veda, a collection of chants intended to promote success, health, and long life. (Practitioners of Ayurveda believe that the sound vibrations from these chants are responsible for their positive effect.) Some ayurvedic healers still use these chants in conjunction with the administration of herbal remedies and other treatments.

Ayurvedic Training

Ayurvedic knowledge has been handed down through generations by skilled practitioners of the craft (called *vaidyas*) who have traditionally trained individual students on an individual basis. Today, however, ayurvedic medicine receives major support from the Indian government, which has helped establish ayurvedic medical colleges throughout the country.

In addition to the 50,000 or so formally trained ayurvedic doctors, there are perhaps as many as 200,000 "unregistered" practitioners with no officially recognized training. In that respect, ayurvedic medicine is not only the major, official form of medical practice in India but it is also the primary form of folk healing. Two less widely practiced forms of folk healing are the *Unani* and *Siddha* medical systems.

Music therapy also plays a part in ayurvedic medicine. It is thought to eliminate imbalances in the body that cause ill health.

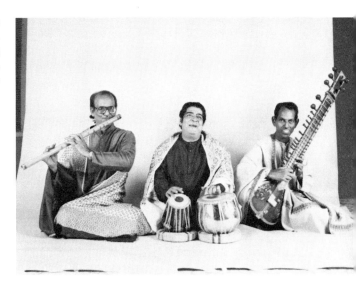

Principles of Ayurveda

According to the ayurvedic system, five primary elements, or *bhutas*—earth, water, light, air, and ether—make up both the universe and the human body. Various combinations of these elements make up the seven tissues, or *dhatus*, of ayurvedic medicine: plasma, blood, muscle, fat, bone, marrow (the soft tissue inside bones), and semen. The body's waste products—urine, sweat, and hair—are termed *malas*.

Doshas

Humans are thought to have different physical attributes (including strength, weakness, and sensitivity to cold or to certain foods) depending upon the relative amounts of three substances, called *doshas*, each person possesses. The three doshas are: *vata*, or air; *pitta*, or fire; and *kapha*, or water.

Disease and Balance

As in traditional Chinese medicine, an important aspect of ayurvedic diagnosis is examination of the patient's pulse. This technique has reached a high degree of sophistication in ayurvedic medicine, in which different characteristics of the pulse—such as frequency and intensity—are believed to reflect the state of internal organs, reveal illness, and indicate imbalances in the doshas.

Diseases and other physical problems are thought to occur when the doshas are not in their proper proportions. It is believed, for example, that a person with too much vata suffers from excessive worrying and fear and talks, eats, and walks quickly. This person's pulse is said to be irregular, or "crooked." Among bodily ailments thought to be caused by an imbalance of vata are asthma, constipation, some headaches, backaches, and sexual problems.

Someone with a pitta personality, on the other hand, is very active and intelligent but is also likely to express anger and hate and to suffer

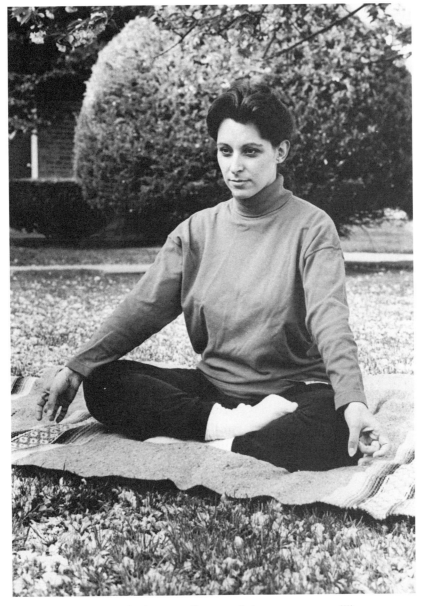

Yoga serves as a sort of preventive medicine; many practitioners believe that it helps the body and mind maintain a state of balance and can be used to head off the onset of disease.

from such disorders as ulcers, hemorrhoids, and migraine headaches. A kapha person tends to be self-controlled, mild, stable, and patient but may also be possessive and greedy. This person tends to be overweight and to have a slow pulse.

Treatment Strategies of Ayurveda

Rather than treating symptoms, ayurvedic doctors attempt to cure an illness permanently by trying to enhance the body's own disease-fighting immune system through diet and medicine.

Ayurveda contends that foods contain the essences of each dosha—air, fire, and water—although usually one dosha dominates the others. Therefore, an ayurvedic physician would choose to give or withhold from a patient particular types of food, depending upon the patient's state. For example, if a patient had high fever and thirst, a physician might prescribe "water" foods, such as lemons, grapefruits, and pears.

Treating Simple and Complex Diseases

The common cold is familiar to patients around the world. In India, a vaidya might prescribe herbal tea, fluids, rest, and perhaps an alteration of daily routines to avoid aggravating the condition—a treatment not all that different from one prescribed by many American grandmothers.

However, the ayurvedic treatment of diabetes, a potentially fatal disease in which the body cannot effectively transfer sugar from the blood to the cells to use as an energy source, demonstrates the important fine points of this form of folk healing. A vaidya would tell his diabetic patient to avoid starchy foods, sweet fruits, and sugar in any form. In addition, the physician would concoct any of several preparations to reduce the level of sugar in the blood. One of these formulations, a *dhanvantari ghrita*, is an assortment of plant juices dissolved or suspended in *ghee* (boiled, purified butter). The ghrita is given orally or applied to the skin, and its *lipoidal* (fatty) characteristics help the body absorb and use the sugar-lowering ingredients. In recent years, laboratory experiments have demonstrated that some of the plants con-

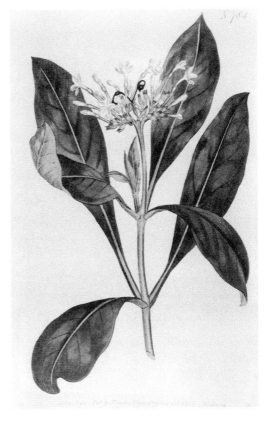

Snakeroot, used for centuries by Indian healers to calm mentally disturbed patients, contains the ingredient reserpine, now a medication used by Western physicians to control high blood pressure.

tained in this drug really do have hypoglycemic activity and can reduce blood sugar levels.

In all, there are hundreds of plants that find use in ayurvedic medicine, some of which have been systematically studied by researchers in order to discover how they produce their effects. As these studies continue, the value of ayurvedic medicine will be better appreciated and the healing power of plants will be better understood.

Ayurvedic drugs are meticulously prepared according to a *formulary*—a collection of "recipes" for making medicinal preparations —that is published by the Indian government. The formulary directs how to blend and process roots, fruit pulp, seeds, stems, and other plant parts to make various medicines.

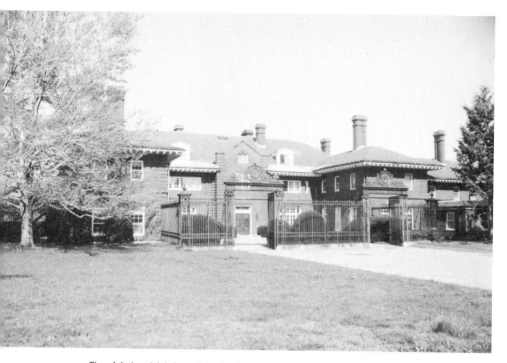

The Maharishi Ayur-Veda Center for Stress Management and Behavioral Medicine in Lancaster, Massachusetts; there has been a growing appreciation in the United States for the potential healing power of Indian folk medicine.

Bhasmas: Medication Without Plants

The *bhasmas*, another group of ayurvedic preparations, contain metals rather than plants and occasionally marine and animal products as well. The diabetes medication, *trivanga bhasma*, for example, contains equal proportions of lead, tin, and zinc. The *loha bhasma* preparation, which contains iron, is used to treat anemia as well as diabetes, and the *vang bhasma*, which contains tin, is used to treat asthma.

Other forms of therapy used in ayurvedic practice include exposure to sunlight, exercise, enemas, bloodletting, and laxatives. Muscle massage is also widely used and is performed following the application of herbal oil to the skin's surface.

YOGA: MIND OVER BODY

Yoga (derived from the Sanskrit word meaning "union") is a general term for the spiritual disciplines designed to help an individual attain higher consciousness, liberation from ignorance and suffering, and rebirth as a newer, better person. Like ayurvedic medicine, the practice of yoga—with its familiar, cross-legged position; its practitioner sitting and silently meditating—is steeped in ancient religious philosophy.

The aim of yoga as a medical discipline is to help the body and mind maintain a state of balance in the face of various problems, such as physical illness or psychological stress. But yoga therapy does not exclude medical treatment of disease. In fact, many *yogins* (practitioners of yoga) use herbal and ayurvedic remedies for such purposes.

In general, yoga stresses the spiritual lift one attains from good hygiene and proper health measures—not just freedom from disease, but an energetic feeling of well-being that translates into overall health and resistance to disease. In other words, yoga is meant to serve as *preventive medicine*, to head off the onset of disease rather than to eradicate ill health. Indeed, the correct practice of yoga has been shown to reduce such symptoms of stress as *hypertension* (high blood pressure). This may be of particular concern in underdeveloped countries, where *tranquilizing* (calming) medication is either too expensive or not available.

EASTERN MEDICINE IN THE UNITED STATES

Just as some elements of traditional Chinese medicine have found their way to the United States, the same holds true for Indian folk healing. For example, Indian vaidyas have used the powdered root of the *snakeroot* plant for centuries to calm mentally disturbed patients. Western physicians began using the powder's active ingredient, *reserpine*, in 1953, finding it useful for the same purpose and also utilizing its ability to reduce dangerously high blood pressure. Although newer medications have replaced reserpine in psychiatric treatment, this ancient medicine is still used to control blood pressure in the West.

The growing appreciation in the United States for the potential healing power of Indian folk medicine was also demonstrated, as previously mentioned, by the weekend training session in ayurvedic medicine held in 1987 in Lancaster, Massachusetts. By 1988, Ayurveda-trained physicians were administering herbal treatments and massage to patients at ayurvedic centers in Lancaster, Massachusetts; Fairfield, Iowa; Palm Beach, Florida; Washington, D.C.; and Pacific Palisades, California.

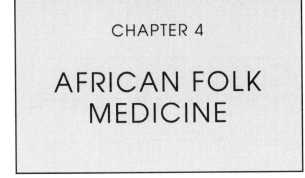

CHAPTER 4

AFRICAN FOLK MEDICINE

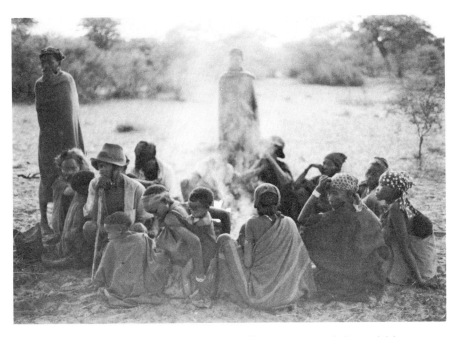

A !Kung bushman healing dance; the ceremony is thought to enhance the curing powers of bushman trance healers.

Bushman medicine is put into the body through the backbone. It boils in my belly and boils up to my head like beer. When the women start singing and I start dancing, at first I feel quite all right. Then in the middle, the medicine begins to rise from my stomach. . . . You feel your blood become very hot just like blood boiling on a fire and then you start healing. . . . The thing comes up after a dance, then when I lay hands on a sick person, the medicine in me will go into him and cure him.

This colorful, personal account of a !Kung Bushman *trance healer* (the exclamation point stands for the characteristic click sound that is part of the !Kung language) was published in *Natural History* magazine in 1967. The description illustrates a concept critical to much traditional healing in Africa: the connection between the healer and the higher power to which the healer appeals on behalf of a patient.

Despite the introduction of modern medicine in Africa, these folk practitioners continue to thrive, mostly because newer techniques are unavailable to much of the population. Even when a small Western-style medical facility does exist in a rural area, many Africans will seek help from a folk healer as well. Thus, traditional healers still tend to the needs of more than half of the population of Africa.

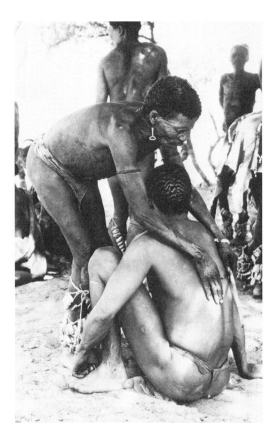

After entering a trance, a !Kung healer attempts to treat a patient.

Another important reason for the tenacity of African folk medicine is that its roots, like that of Chinese and ayurvedic medicine, are deeply embedded in the rich and varied traditions of the numerous African tribes. Both culture and religion play important roles in the traditional African concepts of disease and healing.

Therefore, folk doctors offer more than the hope of a cure. Unlike modern physicians, these healers possess the same traditional views of illness and treatment as their patients do. For example, germs and parasites are not part of the traditional understanding of disease processes in Africa. Rather, many individuals—healers and patients alike—believe that magical spells or angry spirits are responsible for illness. Traditional healers tend to respond to a patient's questions concerning these mystical sources more sympathetically than do Western-trained physicians, and they are more attuned to the healing power of herbs than are modern doctors. Thus, common perspectives forge links between patients and folk healers that are far stronger than those between modern doctors and their patients.

Even in those cases in which modern medicine is available and is the only hope for patients, a lack of education and rampant superstition leave many Africans unequipped to make informed decisions about whether to take advantage of it. Therefore, the old ways of healing are the only ways that many Africans are comfortable with.

A folk doctor's expertise does not come easily, however. In many cases, an African healer's training begins very early in childhood and lasts a lifetime. The instruction can include lessons taught by and observation of an established healer, supervised healing, and at times temporary solitude in the forest, where the young healer meditates, communes with nature, and perhaps even undergoes self-torture and self-denial of comforts.

DIAGNOSIS AND TREATMENT

Like Western physicians, many traditional African healers conduct a careful diagnosis. Although techniques differ from one culture to another, the exam often begins with the healer obtaining a history of the disease from the patient, followed by a physical checkup. Folk

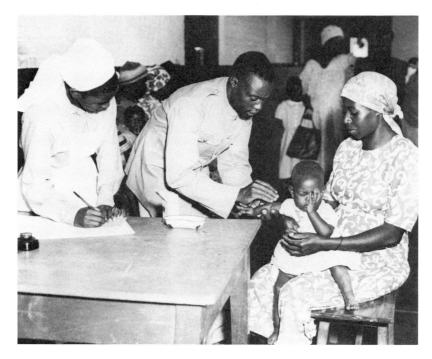

Despite the spread of Western medicine throughout Africa, such as at this clinic in Rhodesia (1955), traditional healing remains an important part of health care.

healers may, for example, tap on different parts of the body looking for tender spots, feel the heartbeat, and check the eyes and ears.

Once a problem is diagnosed, the healer typically prescribes herbal medicines and, during a recuperation period at home (or at the home of the healer), family members and friends visit the patient to offer support and encouragement.

Yet despite the pride that traditional healers generally take in their profession, they frequently desire collaboration with Western-trained physicians working nearby and sometimes refer their own patients to them as well. Such collaboration often adds to the arsenal of curative techniques learned by the folk healer. Similarly, the wisdom of traditional African healers—especially their knowledge of the healing power of plants—is coming under greater scrutiny by scientists.

HEALING BODY AND MIND

Lacking such Western "necessities" as aspirin, laxatives, and other over-the-counter drugs and ready-made prescription medications, African folk healers nevertheless have tended to their patients' medical needs for centuries. In addition, many healers play additional roles such as marital counselor and child psychologist and are looked to by all members of their society—from peasants to leaders—for advice, treatments, and cures.

The power of the medicines that traditional healers administer is apparently enhanced by the *placebo effect* (in which a medical treatment works because the patient believes it will, not because the treatment itself is inherently valuable). Patients may be instructed to wear a *curative object*, perhaps a bone or stone that is believed to possess power against sickness. The individual's belief in that object proves reassuring and helps him or her feel better. Such objects are used for a variety of ailments, including headaches, malaria, stomachaches, lunacy, and sexual impotency.

DIVINERS

Perhaps no other type of healer so aptly reflects the religious origins of his or her healing powers than the *diviner*, a religious-medical specialist who not only diagnoses a patient's illness but also determines its cause by means of contact with superhuman or spiritual sources. *Divination*, then, is reminiscent of the powers attributed to the oracles of ancient Greece, who were thought to be able to foretell events through their connection with supernatural powers.

The African diviner is considered to be the one person in the community who is closest to God, according to Dr. F. M. Mburu in the book *Traditional Healing: New Science or New Colonialism?* As such, the diviner is capable of understanding spiritual and supernatural phenomena. Thus, he or she is usually highly respected and is called upon not only to cure various ills—such as stomach disorders, headaches, infectious diseases, skin diseases, and wounds—but also to give advice to people in the community.

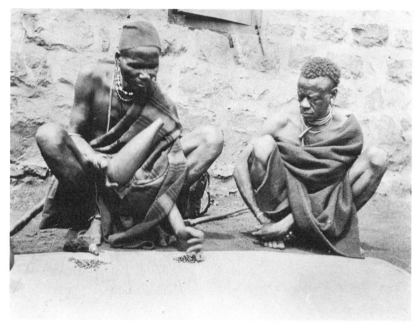

In Africa, diviners are believed capable of diagnosing an illness through contact with superhuman or spiritual forces. Here a diviner from Kenya attempts to gain insight into a patient's illness using seeds, pebbles, and other objects poured from a special gourd.

In addition, some African cultures believe that illness and misfortune can result from being cursed. An evil diviner, or witch doctor, is believed to be able to cast such a spell at the request of a client wishing to harm an enemy. An important element of a diviner's reputation is his or her supposed ability to break curses cast by others.

Although there is often competition between modern physicians and traditional healers, Mburu found during his studies of traditional medicine in Kenya that diviners sometimes refer their patients to hospitals when necessary and that these diviners sometimes make use of Western-trained physicians themselves when they contract "European diseases"—diseases that are unknown to them.

TRADITIONAL HEALING
AMONG THE BAMBARA

It is difficult to describe folk medicine in Africa in broad, sweeping terms. Yet the Bambara tribes of the Republic of Mali in West Africa, who are served by a wide variety of traditional healers, provide a good representative look at folk medicine customs practiced throughout much of the continent. This great diversity in the healing arts used throughout Africa was documented through eyewitness accounts by Dr. Pascal James Imperato in his book *African Folk Medicine*.

Folk Specialists

Bonesetters, naturally, specialize in treating patients with broken bones. Fractures can often heal themselves, and in such cases merely wrapping the limb and telling the patient to be careful with it are enough to ensure recovery.

Surgery, another specialty, is also commonly performed, but it is guided by traditional rituals rather than by modern techniques. A Bambara surgeon typically uses either knives or razors to make a few parallel incisions over the affected area of the body while performing a ritual chant. After making the cuts, the traditional surgeon commonly performs a procedure known as *cupping*. In this procedure, the healer places the wide end of a cow horn over the incision and sucks out the air through a hole in the tip, thus creating a vacuum, according to Imperato's account.

Often the surgeon will place a piece of beeswax over the hole in order to maintain the vacuum for up to half an hour. (Imperato also reported having observed some healers in Tanzania who would place a substance in their mouth before sucking on the horn and then spitting the material out, telling the patient that the substance had come out of the incision.)

Herbalists, in contrast, use their well-established list of plant preparations—often simply passed from parent to child by word of mouth—

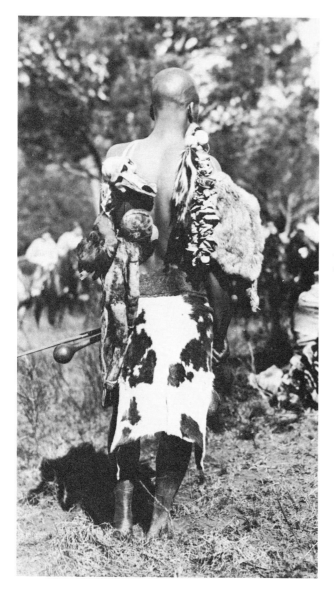

A healer from South Africa's Fish River Tribe displays two magic charms: a baboon skull and a stuffed monkey.

to treat illnesses. But their knowledge of poisonous plants also gives these healers a potential dark side: Among the Bambara, herbalists sometimes provide deadly plants to clients, who slip these poisons into the food of their enemies.

Like the bonesetter, the herbalist does not necessarily face criticism if patients are not "cured" according to Western standards. Rather than attributing failure to deficient herbs or bad technique, the problem may be interpreted by the patient or the herbalist as being the result of supernatural forces or witchcraft. In such cases, the patient may turn to a diviner for help.

THE HEALING DANCE

Herbs and divination are considered powerful healing tools by many Africans. But dance, as seen in the case of the !Kung Bushmen, is at least as powerful—and ancient—as any other medicine or healing art. This technique reflects the view of traditional Africans that there is continuous interaction between spiritual forces and the community. Dancing is one way to imitate, appeal to, or appease these forces on behalf of the welfare of the individual.

Among the Jukun people of Nigeria, for example, folk practitioners may try to heal female tribe members by performing an *exorcism* (a ritual conducted to rid the body of evil spirits) during initiation ceremonies. The sufferer learns songs and dances that have therapeutic value and then joins a public ceremony to perform the ritual initiation dance.

On the other hand, the healing dances of the Yoruba people in southwestern Nigeria pay homage to Shango, the god of thunder and lightning. The Shango priest, who is thought by believers to become possessed during the dance, enters a deep trance, during which the healer expresses Shango's wrath by performing both lightning-quick movements of the arms and powerful shoulder rolls. During the 19th century, Shango was exported to the West Indies island of Trinidad, where it became mixed with various tenets of Catholicism.

SNAKE CULTS

The widespread fear of poisonous snakes in Africa has given rise to a group of healing specialists who treat snakebites. Members of secret societies called *snake cults* claim to be capable of making their clients

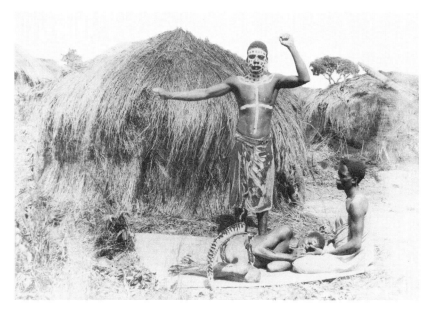

An African folk doctor makes healing gestures over his patient. A water buck's horn containing medicine has been placed over the diseased area.

immune to snakebites and to be able to cure them of poisoning if they are bitten.

Cult members learn how to capture and handle pythons, green mambas, gabon vipers, and other dangerous snakes, come to know their habits, and are taught how to treat snakebites. In Liberia, for example, cult members chew the leaves of the *Microdesmis puberula* tree and spit out the shredded, wet pulp onto the snake's head. A substance released when the leaves are chewed makes the snake lethargic and easy to handle.

The actual treatment of snakebites varies from place to place. In Liberia, cult members combine buds of the plant *Dichrostachys glomerata* with white clay and rub the mixture into the wounds made by the bite of the green mamba. To treat black cobra bites, the healer first puts the buds of a plant from the genus *Mezoneurom* in his or her mouth, then sucks the victim's wound. Afterward, a mixture of white clay and beaten leaves of *Similax kraussiana* is applied to the wound. The active ingredients used in these treatments render at least some snakebite remedies successful.

BAD MAGIC

Despite the proliferation of folk medicine practitioners working to improve health and relieve discomfort, some members of African communities specialize in attempting to harm others—for a fee. These *sorcerers* (who are somewhat different from witch doctors) are believed to know the secrets of "bad magic," which involves the use of herbs, hair, or other objects over which they have chanted secret words. Deposited near the victim's doorway, hidden in or near his or her house, or placed under the bed, these objects are believed to be able to bring harm—including illness—to that person.

Although sorcerers are generally men, women—in the form of witches—are also thought to play a role in evil magic and ill health. Unlike sorcerers, witches are considered to possess their malicious powers from birth and may not even realize that they have such abilities. A witch traditionally evokes more fear and hatred among Africans than a sorcerer does, because she is thought to be a continuous threat to the souls and health of people in whatever village she lives. In response, women thought to be witches have often been tortured and killed.

Such drastic action is less common today, but fear of witches, sorcerers, and evil spirits in general is still widespread. In fact, it is still customary for people who fall ill to accuse specific individuals of having used evil magic or of having hired a sorcerer to cause the illness.

Protection from Evil

Some diviners give their patients *amulets*—small handmade or found objects believed to be endowed with special healing or protective powers—to shield them from the danger of witches and sorcerers. These amulets, which may be stones, claws, animal teeth, or lockets, are thought to derive their powers from natural or religious forces. Other healing and protective objects, called *talismans*, bear signs or engraved characters and are thought to act as charms to avert evil and bring good fortune.

PLANT PRESCRIPTIONS

Although many herbal remedies are common throughout much of Africa, the name of a particular plant may vary from one tribe to another. For example, *Alstonia boonei*, a member of the dogbane family of flowering plants, is called *Sinduru* by residents of the Ivory Coast, *Bokuka* in Zaire, and *Myna* in Uganda. The use of these plants can also differ from one area to another.

Tribal healers perform during a welcoming ceremony in the township of Soweto for South African freedom fighter Nelson Mandela, following his release from prison in February 1990.

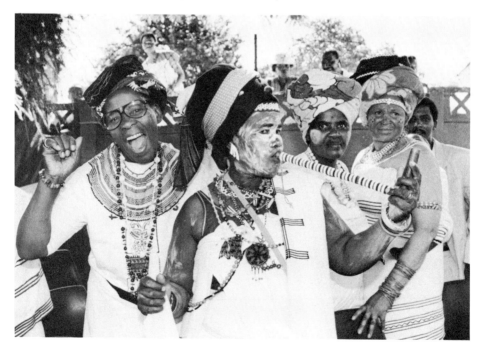

A. boonei, which is found mostly in lowland forests and wet, marshy areas, is widely distributed in northern tropical Africa (Senegal, Guinea, the Ivory Coast, Nigeria, and Uganda). *A. boonei* is a large tree that bears fruit from December to May. An *infusion* of stem bark (produced by soaking the bark in hot or cold water to extract its active ingredients) is drunk by some people to cure worms or snakebite, to relax muscles, or as a cure for rheumatic pains. An infusion of bark and leaves is drunk as an asthma remedy.

The bark of another tree, the West African *Anthocleista nobilis*, is boiled with water and the extract taken once a day for intestinal problems. In the Central African Republic, the bark is used to promote bowel movements, as an antidote for poison, and as a treatment for leprosy.

Altogether, there are probably hundreds of plants that are part of the healing traditions of African tribes. Western scientists, including those from the World Health Organization (which is part of the United Nations) and private drug companies, are currently studying many of these plants in order to discover new medicines.

HERBALISM'S STRONG HOLD

During the 19th century, European colonialists in Africa attempted to eradicate "primitive" beliefs in such matters as local religions and herbalism, according to a report by Joseph O. Lambo in the book *Traditional Healing: New Science or New Colonialism?*

Colonial authorities often harassed herbalists and accused them of injuring their patients. African healers have resisted this relentless effort to erase their heritage in a struggle that has persisted into the 20th century. For example, in 1947, the *Nigerian Association of Medical Herbalists* was established to revitalize the profession of herbalism and to convince the government of Nigeria that this form of healing deserves support. Under the leadership of its third president, the afore-mentioned Joseph Lambo, the association helped persuade Nigerian scientists to study the healing powers of herbs. Other organizations, such as the *Herbalists' Association of Malawi*, also continue to preserve the rich heritage of this form of African folk healing.

Thus, despite the slow but relentless spread of Western medicine throughout Africa, herbalists today remain firmly entrenched in their society. The continuing hold that traditional healers have on much of the African population reflects the deep-rooted mystical beliefs held by many Africans concerning the cause and cure of illness. In response, the government of Zimbabwe encouraged the foundation of that country's traditional healers' association, which attempts to regulate healers and discourage the practice of witchcraft. The association also affords the government an opportunity to encourage traditional healers to use some modern therapies when necessary.

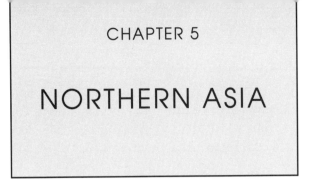

CHAPTER 5

NORTHERN ASIA

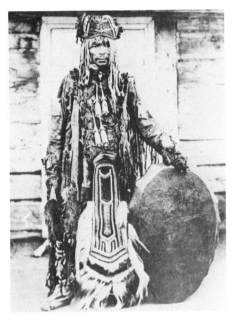

A Tungus shaman from northern Siberia; the shaman serves as a healer and diviner, as well as an escort to the afterlife for the souls of the dead.

Flickering flames throw eerie shadows on the walls of a tent that shuts out the frigid Siberian winter. A mysterious figure, wearing a crown of antlers and dressed in a deerskin coat fringed with leather ribbons, lifts his head heavenward. He raises a wooden drumstick that is decorated with animal and human figures and begins to strike his fur-covered, animal-skin drum. Accompanied by the haunting, thumping rhythm of the drum, this extraordinary being begins to dance around the fire.

Lulled into a state of ecstasy by the beating of the drum and empowered by the spirits that have entered his body, the figure sings an improvised song filled with metaphors, images, and dialogue. It is a song that tells the breathless spectators of his voyage to the "other side," to the realm of the spirits.

As his assistant feeds the fire, the figure continues his performance, dancing to the rhythm of the thumping drum and the jingling of trinkets hanging from his robe. The observers come to believe that the healer-diviner they are watching, a shaman, is capable of curing any illness, foretelling the future, and communicating with spirits.

SHAMANISM

The shaman's profession, *shamanism*, consists primarily of traditional religious and healing customs found in Siberia and other parts of northern Asia. According to "The Shaman and the Medicine-Man," a scholarly comparison of these two forms of healing by Ake Hultkrantz, published in *Social Science and Medicine* (1985), the word *shaman* is derived from the language of the Tungus people of Siberia. Hultkrantz defines the shaman as "a social functionary who, with the help of guardian spirits, attains ecstasy in order to create a rapport with the supernatural world on behalf of his group members." The more literal meaning for the term *shaman* is simply "he who knows."

Ancient Roots of Shamanism

Shamanism stretches back to the days of prehistoric hunter-gatherer societies. The shaman actually is a healer, a diviner, and a *psychopomp* (someone who escorts the souls of the dead to the afterlife). As such, he is a revered, sometimes feared, figure, who can induce a state of ecstasy within himself on behalf of his client. (The term *ecstasy* is derived from the Greek word *ekstasis*, meaning: "to stand outside of, or transcend, oneself." The primary goal of ecstasy is to experience an inner vision of God or of one's relation to or union with a divine spirit.)

Since the ability to fall into a trancelike state of ecstasy is found in people throughout the world, the essential features that produce a true shaman are the beliefs, actions, mystical objects, clothing, and rites connected with the ecstatic state.

The Making of a Shaman

Although the shaman is held in high esteem and supported by the community so that the healer does not have to engage in common labor for food and clothing, the road to becoming a shaman is not normally one that successful candidates choose for themselves. Instead, individuals are chosen by the "spirits" to follow the calling.

Often, the chosen one is somehow different from others in the community. Perhaps the individual has more fingers or toes, suffers from epilepsy (a brain disorder that causes seizures), or actually has a

An Alaskan folk healer; although the classic shamans are found in Siberia and other parts of northern Asia, the Inuit and the peoples of Southeast Asia do have shamanlike healers of their own.

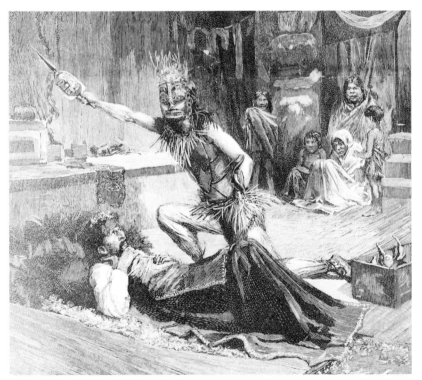

mental illness. What may be considered a physical or psychological problem in the West, then, may well be cherished as the sign of a future shaman in a primitive, rural community in northern Asia.

THE ROLE OF THE SHAMAN

The community calls upon the shaman for assistance during life's great events: birth, marriage, and death. For example, depending upon the tribe, a shaman may ascend to heaven to obtain an embryo soul for a childless woman or may perform rites after the child's birth to keep the infant from crying or to help the baby develop. Some shamans catch the souls of the deceased that float in the universe and escort them to the Yonder World.

Shaman as Healer

When a person falls ill, the shaman may decide the nature of the sacrifice to be made in order to appease the angry spirits who caused the illness. As a result, the patient may have to kill a reindeer or perform some other ritual to regain his or her health.

Among some tribes, illness is thought to be caused by the loss of a person's soul into the hands of spirits who torment it. The shaman's job is to retrieve the soul from these spirits. In other cases, illness is believed to be caused by spirits entering into the patient, so the shaman cures the victim by using special powers to drive out the spirit.

SHAMANLIKE FIGURES OF OTHER CULTURES

Although the healers of Siberia represent the classic example of shamanism, other cultures—including the Alaskan Inuit and the peoples of Southeast Asia—do have shamanlike figures. Inuit shamans, for example, perform healing rituals, as well as ecstatic "underwater" journeys to the Mother of Animals spirit in order to assure an abundance of game. Like the shamans of northern Asia, Inuit shamans also aid in the conception of children.

CHAPTER 6

LATIN AMERICAN FOLK MEDICINE

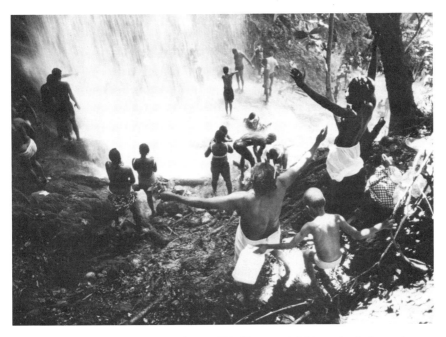

A Voodoo ceremony. A mixture of Haitian and African beliefs and Roman Catholic ritual, Voodoo is a religious and healing cult.

The vision that Mark Plotkin had while sleeping inside his jungle hut in Suriname, South America, threw him into a cold sweat. A jaguar stalked into the hut, strode up to his hammock, and stared into the face of this startled Harvard University scientist. When Plotkin awoke, he was frightened, unsure whether the vision of the jaguar had been a dream or whether he had actually been face-to-face with the wild jungle cat.

The next day Plotkin told the story to the folk healer who had been teaching him the medicinal secrets of South American plants. Until now the healer's disposition had been sour; he suspected that the American scientist did not respect him or his powers. Upon hearing of the scientist's dream that a jaguar had entered the hut, however, the healer smiled and said, "That was me."

Like many others in his profession, the folk doctor claimed to be able to turn himself into a jaguar. The American's vision, the healer thought, had proved to the foreigner that the doctor was worthy of respect.

This story, recounted in the magazine *International Wildlife* (May-June 1984), reflects the intense pride that native healers of the Amazon take in their knowledge of the curative powers of plants and demonstrates the dedication of scientists like Mark Plotkin, who spend years living in primitive, tropical areas to further the study of medicinal plant use by primitive tribes.

These researchers collect and examine plants that local herbalists in Mexico, Central America, and South America claim have the power to cure various illnesses. Plotkin's predecessor from Harvard, for example, Richard Evans Schultes, was a giant in the field of plant medicines. Working in the Amazon jungle from 1941 to 1954, Schultes suffered through mosquitoes, hunger, and disease to study the ways of jungle healers and to collect about 24,000 plants previously unknown

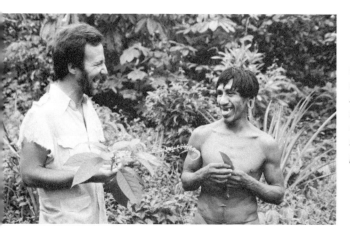

Mark Plotkin, pictured here with a South American Indian folk healer, is a Harvard University scientist who studies the medicinal power of plants.

to the developed world. South American Indians use more than 1,300 of these plants in some way—often as medicines.

MEDICINAL PLANTS

A seemingly ordinary fruit, the avocado, has a long history of medicinal use in Latin America, and several different species grow throughout the region. Healers in Mexico use oil extracted from the seeds of the *Persea americana* avocado to treat dysentery, and the skin of the avocado fruit is used to fight infections of the skin as well as digestive ailments.

In Brazil, the resin of the flowering shrub called Incense of America (*Styrax camporum*) is used either externally as a germ-killing (antiseptic) soap to treat skin disease or internally to treat digestive illnesses, including ulcers.

In Mexico, the flower of the evergreen tree *Talauma mexicana* is so renowned for its use as a folk treatment for heart ailments that

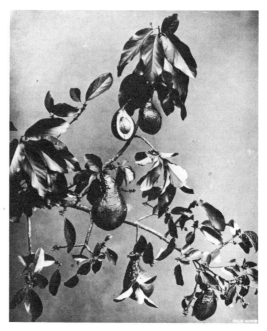

The avocado has a long history as a Latin American folk medicine; its use includes treatment of skin infections and dysentery.

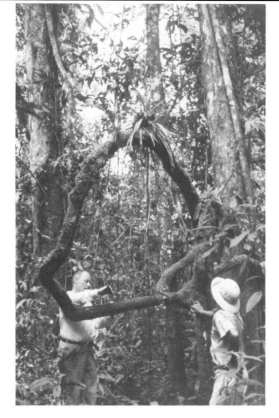

The Chondodendron tomentosum *vine, from which the poison curare is derived; curare was adopted by Western physicians for use as a muscle relaxant for surgical patients.*

Mexico's National Institute of Cardiology uses the plant as part of its symbol. At least one scientific study, in fact, has shown that *Talauma* can indeed stimulate the heart.

Curare, an extract derived from either the *Chondodendron tomentosum* or the *Strychnos toxifera* vines in the Amazon, where natives used it to make poison arrows, was adopted by Western physicians as a muscle relaxant for patients undergoing complicated surgery. Sap from a tree of the nutmeg family has long been used to treat fungal infections of the skin by natives in such areas as the northwest Amazon, Suriname, and Brazil. When chemists examined the sap, they found three new compounds with fungus-fighting capabilities.

By the 1980s, scientists at the *Beneficial Plant Research Association* in Arizona were actively studying a variety of plants used by traditional Latin American healers, including the bark of *Brunfelsia grandiflora*, which is used by folk doctors to treat arthritis, and the sap of the Amazonian tree, *Croton*, which stimulates wound healing.

In addition, the World Health Organization, the World Wildlife Fund, and the International Union for the Conservation of Nature and Natural Resources are all encouraging scientists to study the medicinal powers of plants.

In spite of this, however, relatively few researchers are following up leads in trying to find active ingredients in the saps, barks, leaves, and fruits of Latin America. Moreover, with tens of thousands of plant species to study, *ethnobotanists* (scientists who study the plant lore of a group or race of people) are in a battle against time. Folk healers with an extensive knowledge of these plants are not being replaced as rapidly as they die. Their traditions—and much potentially valuable knowledge—are dying with them. Moreover, civilization is encroaching farther and farther into the Amazon rainforest. As more and more trees are cut down for lumber or to make way for profitable cattle pastures, potentially valuable species of plants may be vanishing in the process.

TRADITIONAL CURES REFLECT LOCAL DISEASES

As with folk cures everywhere, the most commonly used treatments in a local area generally reflect the specific diseases that often afflict that local population.

For example, in the rural highland area of the Central American country of Guatemala, many plant medicines are used to treat digestive ailments, according to "Digestive Disorders and Plant Medicinals in Highland Guatemala," a report in the book *Health and the Human Condition* (1978). In fact, diseases that cause diarrhea (which can result in severe dehydration) are the major cause of death in Guatemala.

DEADLY CONSEQUENCES OF SOME TRADITIONAL BELIEFS

The evolution of traditional medicine occurred within the various cultural and religious frameworks of Latin American countries, and it has fulfilled the needs of people faced with both routine and life-

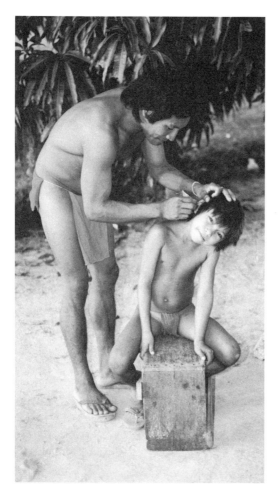

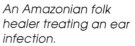

An Amazonian folk healer treating an ear infection.

threatening diseases but who have few medical resources except the healing plants of the jungles. In some cases, however, particular beliefs have proved fatal.

For example, some highland parents in rural Guatemala attempt to cure diarrhea by severely restricting the amount of food and water their sick child consumes. Instead of solidifying the child's stools, however, the treatment only aggravates the dehydration caused by diarrhea. Rather than curing the children, the treatment often kills them.

HALLUCINOGENS AND HEALING

Hallucinogenic substances have also become an important part of Latin American healing techniques. Indians of the Orinoco and Amazon regions of South America commonly drink a concoction called *aya-huasca* (or *yage*), which is produced from the stem bark of the climbing, woody vine *Banisteriopsis caapi*. The Indians believe the drink has curative powers. Although usually restricted to use by healers, Indians of the Uaupes River area in northern Brazil utilize ayahuasca as an essential part of their religious festivals. In the northern Amazon area, Indians inhale a form of snuff called *yopo*, a powerful hallucinogen derived from the *Piptadenia peregrina* tree.

Mushrooms and Other Psychedelic Substances

Long considered to be only legend by scientists, plants such as sacred, hallucinogenic mushrooms and a species of morning glory that causes intoxication became objects of intense interest after botanist Richard Schultes discovered them being used by shamans in Oaxaca, a state in southern Mexico.

The chief species of hallucinogenic mushrooms used in Mexico is *Psilocybe mexicana*, the active chemical of which is *psilocybin*, a substance similar to the compound *D-lysergic acid diethylamide*, or LSD, a drug commonly abused in the United States. So-called magic mushrooms are found throughout Latin American jungles and their use is centuries old. In ancient Guatemala, artists of the Mayan culture in Central America crafted little images in the form of mushrooms.

The Spanish conquerors of the region suppressed the drug-taking cults of the Indians, forcing them into the rural areas of Mexico. They remained hidden there until 1955, when religious scholar R. Gordon Wasson and his companions were invited by Indians to be the first non-Indians to eat sacred mushrooms during a nighttime ceremony. The publicity that followed drew other Americans to the region but also attracted the notice of police, who tried to stop the use of the hal-

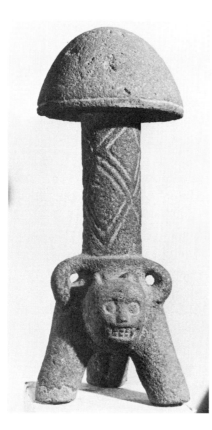

Guatemalan carving of an animal with a mushroom growing from its back. Hallucinogenic mushrooms and other mind-altering substances play an important part in Latin American folk healing.

lucinogen. Today the mushroom cults still exist, yet perform their ceremonies less openly.

Indians in Mexico (as well as in the United States and Canada) also ingest the dried tops of another hallucinogenic plant, the *peyote* cactus, *Lophophora williamsii*. The dried cactus tops contain the chemical *mescaline*, which produces "visions" in those who consume them. Traditional healers in Peru also use psychedelic drugs derived from cactus plants. The ritual preparation and ceremonial use of these psychedelic substances has, over time, come to incorporate many religious traditions imported from Europe and Africa, including prayers, fasting, and the use of alcohol.

HEALING CULTS

Healing rituals in Latin America are not restricted to shamans and herbalists. Throughout South and Central America, formal religious groups, called *healing cults*, focus their faith on the worship of a particular saint or spirit or on the powers of a specific human being thought to have the ability to heal. Generally, the groups operate in shrines or at cult centers, invoking spirits who communicate to the worshipers through a healer. In addition, fragments of religion—especially Roman Catholicism—imported into an area have often become intertwined with the rites and customs of a cult. Healing cults, then, are usually a mixture of religion and magic.

VOODOO

Sometime during the 18th century, slaves brought to Haiti from West Africa by the French to work on the sugar plantations fused their religious and magical beliefs with Roman Catholic rituals, producing a new religious and healing cult: Voodoo. The term *Voodoo* comes from the African word *vodun*, a god or spirit. Vodun is also sometimes used as an alternate name for the cult.

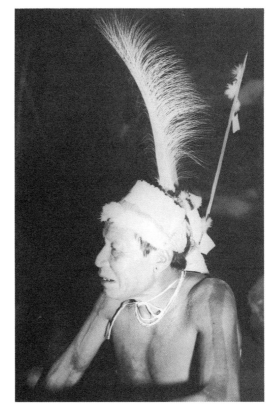

This Colombian Indian medicine man is about to diagnose an ailing young boy; first, however, the healer took a hallucinogen that he believes allows him to talk to the spirits who send disease.

Midnight rendezvous in jungle clearings, animal sacrifices, and dancing women swirling through the night air to the rhythm of drums: These are the images conjured up by outsiders when they think of Voodoo. But the cult is more complex than this. Voodoo rituals involve a mixture of Western religion, Haitian and African beliefs, and drugs.

Voodoo Leaders

Each local Voodoo cult has its own meeting place and a leader—either a male *houngan* or a female *mambo*—who acts as a priest, counselor, healer, and protector against sorcery or witchcraft.

In the classic form of Voodoo, as it originated in Haiti, an individual being initiated into the cult undergoes an elaborate ceremony that may include sacrifices to spirits and seclusion at a Voodoo temple, during which the person is thought to be killed by a spirit and then revived, or reborn.

Voodoo Deities

Although Voodoo apparently involves belief in a god similar to the deity of Western religions, the cult's dramatic rituals are directed toward divinities called *loa*, which include Haitian or African gods,

A worshiper thought to be possessed by a spirit during a Voodoo ceremony in Haiti.

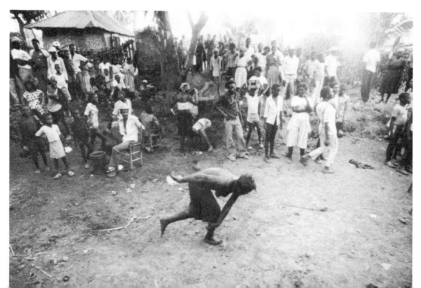

godlike ancestors, and Catholic saints. The loa are guardian angels who communicate with cult members during sleep or during trances brought on during nighttime ritual dancing.

Zombie Potion: Fact or Fiction?

Although various rituals, such as taking sacred mud baths, swimming beneath a sacred waterfall, and animal sacrifice are common among members of Voodoo cults, the most notorious ceremony associated with this religion is *zombification*: turning a person into a *zombie*. Supposedly, a Voodoo sorcerer, called a *bokor*, mixes up a poisonous potion that almost kills the victim. In fact, the individual is thought by others to be dead and is then buried. The bokor later digs up the poisoned individual, revives him or her with an herbal remedy, and keeps the subject in a drugged, passive state.

Wade Davis, a Harvard University ethnobotanist, observed a bokor and his assistants making such a potion. The Voodoo poison makers roast two freshly killed lizards; the carcass of a large, dried and

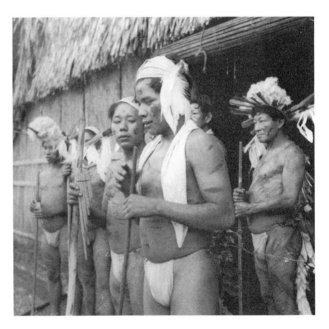

In the Amazon, these young men are preparing for a ceremonial dance, part of an inauguration elevating them to the status of folk healer.

flattened poisonous toad; a sea worm; two sea fish (one of which, the puffer fish, contains a deadly nerve poison called *tetrodotoxin*); and two plants, a legume known locally as *tcha-tcha*, and the "itching pea," which has itch-producing hairs on its seed pod. Two additional—and grotesque—ingredients added are shavings from a human leg bone and the bones of a child, which have been burnt almost to charcoal.

Back in the United States, scientists tested samples of the powder for tetrodotoxin. Some tests found no poison; others found a small amount. Although the popular press spread Davis's belief that tetrodotoxin appeared to be the secret ingredient of zombie powder, much of the scientific community has discounted it. (Davis himself believes that zombification is rare, especially because the amount of tetrodotoxin carried by each puffer fish can vary.)

Moreover, if zombies do exist, they have proved elusive. Western researchers have been able to find only one credible victim, a Haitian man named Clairvius Narcisse. In 1980, 18 years after he had been declared dead, Narcisse returned to his village, claiming to have been enslaved as a zombie. In examining the case, Nathan Kline, a psychiatrist who has spent decades looking into the zombie legend, found Narcisse's story convincing.

CHAPTER 7

CUBAN AND NATIVE AMERICAN FOLK HEALING

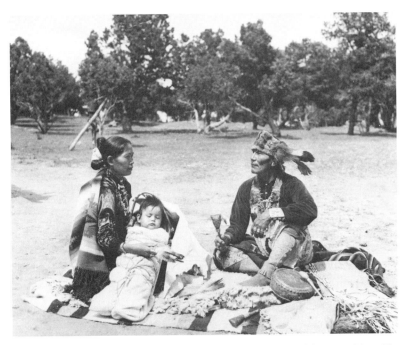

A Navajo medicine man performs a chant to provide good health for a mother and her baby.

Along with the immense variety of folk healing systems found throughout the world, the United States also possesses a rich heritage in traditional medicine. This includes practices imported by immigrants as well as those developed over centuries by Native Americans.

SANTERÍA

Since dictator Fidel Castro's rise to power in Cuba in the 1950s, the influx of refugees from that country to the United States has brought with it a religion combining elements of African and Cuban beliefs. This mixture of magic and Catholicism is called *Santería*.

Origins of Santería

Like Voodoo, Santería has its origins in Africa. It was originally formed centuries ago when Nigerian slaves brought to the New World were introduced to the worship of Catholic saints by their Spanish masters in Cuba and other Latin American nations. Today, Santería, now considered an Afro-Cuban religion, has an elaborate system of rituals and many trained *santeros* and *santeras* (priests and priestesses).

The Draw of Tradition

Santería has especially appealed to those Cuban Americans who feel overwhelmed by the new culture in which they find themselves. The traditional ways of their native country have been challenged by a relatively freewheeling culture of youth, drugs, rock music, and a tendency for both children and women to be much more independent of the family than they were in Cuba.

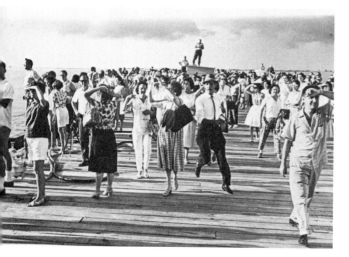

Santería, a religion mixing magic with Catholicism, was brought to the United States by Cuban refugees fleeing the regime of dictator Fidel Castro.

The diminished solidarity of families, a lack of facilities and social clubs catering to Cubans, their inability to speak English, and a sense of political powerlessness in the United States have helped to draw many Cubans to Santería. These immigrants believe that this religion offers a rational explanation for a perceived lack of control over their new life in America and a way to appeal to higher forces for help—help that is often not forthcoming from other, worldly sources.

Santería's Pantheon of Gods

Although there are many different local cults of Santería throughout Latin America and the United States, all share the common worship of the *oricha/santo* (god/saint). There are a number of such gods in Santería, and they are appeased through animal sacrifices or other rituals, such as burning special candles.

The supreme god, *Olodumare-Olofi*, the creator of the universe, is rather remote and generally ignored by Santería priests. His son, *Obatala*, whose Catholic counterpart is Our Lady of Mercy, has great healing powers; if angered, however, he blinds and paralyzes his victims. Thus, these ailments are the ones Santería priests petition him to cure.

Santerían idols

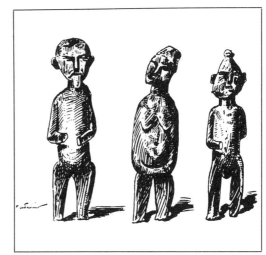

Chango, the passionate oricha and god of thunder, storms, and fire is married to three important goddesses: *Oba*, who some santeros claim rules over bones and cures arthritis and leg paralysis; *Oya*, an aggressive, ill-tempered divinity who controls death; and *Ochun*, the goddess of love and sweet things who controls diseases of the genitals and lower abdomen. In Cuba especially, *Yemaya*, the protector of sailors and fishermen, is considered the mother of all the orichas; in addition, she can cure intestinal ailments as well as tuberculosis. The most feared god of Santería is *Babalu-Aye*, the god of smallpox, syphilis, gangrene, skin ailments, leprosy, and other infectious diseases.

As in other forms of folk healing, the magical and medicinal power of plants play a large role in Santería. Thus, *Osain*, the oricha who presides over flowers, herbs, weeds, twigs, and leaves, must also be appropriately appeased; otherwise, he will destroy their healing powers.

NATIVE AMERICAN
MEDICINE MEN

Like the folk healers of Africa and Latin America, whose traditions have found homes in the United States, the American Indians of North America have a long, proud heritage—and, like their African and Latin American counterparts, American Indian folk healers, often called *medicine men*, have been finding some common ground with modern health care.

Although there are a great variety of medical traditions among the individual tribes across North America, some of the Navajo practices in particular show a number of similarities to folk healing rites of Central and South America.

Among the Navajo, healers use divination to diagnose illness, performing a dramatic, colorful ritual, complete with utterances that reflect supposed possession by spirits. It is assumed, during this rite, that the healer's voice represents that of a god or spirit addressing the patient directly.

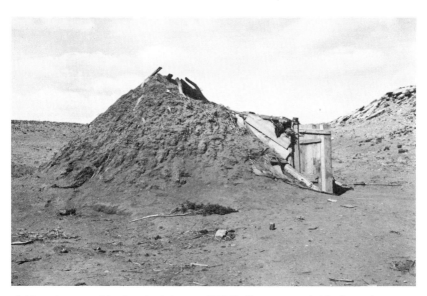

A Navajo sweat lodge in Arizona (1910); these special huts, or hogans, are used in the sweat-emetic purifying ritual.

An herbal treatment of the illness is often undertaken by a separate healer, and one folk practitioner may refer a patient to another if the ailment requires further (or more specialized) care.

Navajo Sweat-emetic Rite

Along with the use of medicinal plants, another Navajo practice consists of purifying the body through a special ritual. The Navajo *sweat-emetic* rite involves cleansing through perspiration as well as through the use of an *emetic*, a substance that causes vomiting.

The ceremony begins with a chanting healer entering a special hut, or *hogan*, accompanied by a procession of individuals seeking to be purified. Once inside, the healer leads the procession in a ritualistic walk around a central fire. An audience of men and women then enters the hut. Next, the chanter heats wooden pokers in the fire; the pokers are applied to the healer's own body (mainly on the legs) and to the people undergoing purification. Following that, the people being purified drink from a basin containing an emetic potion and vomit into receptacles containing sand. Afterward, a *bullroarer* (a heavy stone on a string that makes a roaring noise when twirled) is sounded outside the hut six times. The bullroarer is then brought into the hut and placed over the individuals being purified. The healer's assistants, carrying the basins, lead the audience out of the hogan, while the others remain inside to sweat from the heat of the fire. Once outside, the assistants empty the contents of the receptacles on the ground.

The audience later reenters the hogan, the fire is extinguished, and the healer sprinkles everyone in the tent with a medicinal lotion, fumigating them with incense before they leave once again.

PEYOTE AND THE NATIVE AMERICAN CHURCH

Although to some people, the healing rituals of Native American tribes give fascinating insights into a once-thriving culture, the widespread use of peyote by the Native American Church (a North American Indian religious organization that combines elements of Christianity with Native American beliefs) has evoked not only interest but legal action as well.

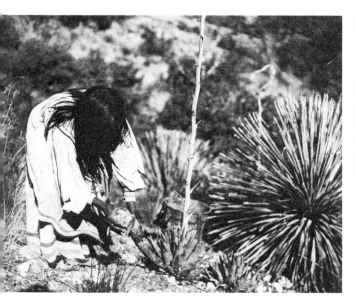

An American Indian woman removing the top of a peyote cactus; widely used by the Native American Church, peyote is believed to enable individuals to commune with a higher world and receive healing power from it.

First used in Mexico about 500 years ago, peyote is an integral part of what is thought to be the most widespread religious movement among North American Indians. Moreover, like the cults of Santería and Voodoo, this movement combines Indian and Christian elements in different degrees, depending upon the particular local form of the religion.

The peyotist doctrine holds that there is one supreme God, the Great Spirit, who communicates with humans through other spirits. In many tribes there is also a Peyote Spirit, who is considered to be either the Indian equivalent of Jesus Christ (the son of God in Christian belief) or to be Jesus Christ himself.

During religious ceremonies, the hallucinations caused by taking peyote are thought to enable individuals to commune with God and the spirits and to receive from them guidance, as well as spiritual and healing power. These ceremonies usually last all night, taking place in a tepee containing a crescent-shaped, earthen altar and a sacred fire. The services, which include prayer, eating of peyote, and several other rituals, are led by a peyote "chief."

Generally, individuals who consume peyote are not prosecuted by the legal authorities of their state; in fact, the federal government and many states with substantial Indian populations have exempted the sacramental use of peyote from criminal penalties. Yet in 1990, a U.S. Supreme Court majority ruled that state governments may prosecute those who use illegal drugs as part of religious rituals without violating their constitutional guarantee of freedom of religion.

Despite the legal wrangling over peyote use, the controversy has not dissuaded anthropologists and even some medical professionals from supporting the practice as an important part of the Native American Church.

In his book *The Dancing Healers—A Doctor's Journey of Healing with Native Americans*, psychiatrist Carl A. Hammerschlag describes his study of Pueblo and Navajo Indian folk medicine. The physician reports that he grew to appreciate the importance the Indians placed on having a feeling of "connectedness" to other people and to the larger community, compared with what he sees as the rush by modern medicine to reduce "healing" to organs, chemical reactions, and drugs.

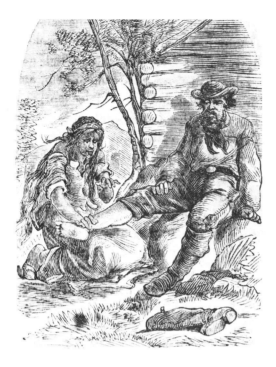

An American Indian woman attempts to cure a case of snakebite with a magic spell.

FOLK HEALERS IN THE HOSPITAL

The "personal touch" of folk healers has made itself felt in hospitals in recent years, as modern physicians have come to understand the great psychological value traditional medicine has to Native American patients. The healing ritual of a medicine man from the Zuni tribe in west-central New Mexico, as described by Scott Camazine of Cornell University in *Folk Medicine: The Art and the Science*, illustrates the treatment of a gunshot wound that had developed an *abscess* (a collection of pus surrounded by inflamed tissue).

The medicine man sat at the bedside of the patient, opened a cornhusk packet filled with white cornmeal, and placed it on the floor. While chanting and moving his hands across the patient's wounded chest, the medicine man produced six small black pebbles and placed them on the cornmeal. These objects, according to the Zuni healer, had been placed on the wound by an enemy to prevent healing.

Although the Zuni know that healers use sleight of hand to accomplish such "cures," this knowledge does not detract from the ritual's ability to ease the patient's anxiety. Rather, because the practices are thought to be sanctioned by the gods, the act symbolizes the healer's relationship with the divinities—and therefore his power to cure.

NATIVE AMERICAN FOLK TRADITIONS FOR SALE

As an increasing number of people have learned to appreciate Native American folk medicine, the demand for information about it has given rise to a thriving business. Books and seminars popularizing Native American culture draw a large audience, and some people, according to a 1988 article in the *Bloomsbury Review*, pay substantial fees to participate in healing rituals and other ceremonies.

Many Native Americans, however, have condemned popular books on Indian customs, claiming that the writers often spread false notions about Native American culture. The critics also insist that sponsors of Indian ceremonies should not be making money by attempting to publicize sacred, ancient rituals.

A Winnebago Indian medicine dance

One such critic, a Sioux scholar, is quoted in the *Bloomsbury Review* article as saying: "The realities of Indian belief and existence have become so misunderstood and distorted at this point that when a real Indian stands up and speaks the truth at any given moment, he or she is not only unlikely to be believed, but will probaby be publicly contradicted and 'corrected' by the citation of some non-Indian and totally inaccurate 'expert.'"

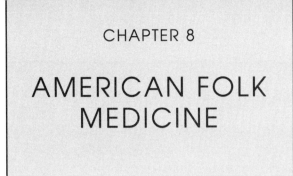

CHAPTER 8

AMERICAN FOLK MEDICINE

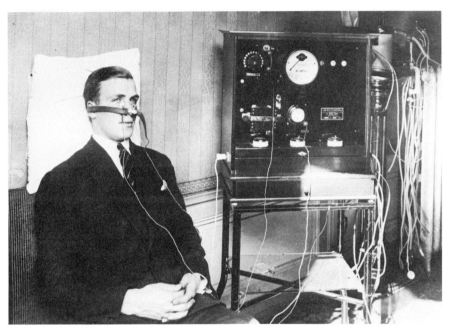

An inventor claimed that this machine could cure the common cold in 10 minutes. Some quack remedies are not just ridiculous but dangerous as well; desperate patients suffering from cancer or AIDS are particularly vulnerable to charlatans.

A long with the rich contributions of Native and Latin Americans, the heritage of immigrants from around the world has also found its way into the folk healing traditions of the United States. Moreover, despite the great amount of costly high-tech medicine available to American citizens, health care based on religious or mystical principles—or on simple remedies handed down from one generation to the next—can still be found today.

In Arkansas, for example, an old man might well teach his grandson to take the plant *mullein* (a plant of the genus *Verbascum*), a popular decongestant in those parts. Up north, in Missouri, one might be lucky enough to meet up with somebody who knows how to make cough syrup from the bark of the wild cherry tree or with an old-timer who uses the white milk squeezed from wild lettuce to cure warts.

The *Charleston Gazette*, a West Virginia newspaper, reported in 1989 that a star athlete on the University of Charleston baseball team found relief from an agonizing muscle ailment in his right shoulder by allowing himself to be stung by bees. Over a 4-week period, the young man received 40 to 50 bee stings and later said that his muscle pain had virtually disappeared. Moreover, he continued to submit to occasional

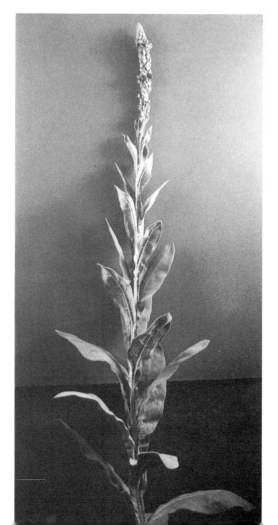

Down South, mullein has been a popular folk remedy for respiratory congestion.

stings to maintain the effect. (If there is any medical validity to this treatment, it apparently lies in the body's supposed release of a painkilling substance that counteracts the bee sting poison.)

HEALING BASED ON SUPERSTITION

Crossroads

An important aspect of many types of folk medicine is the belief that the charms or spells will work only if the ritual is performed in the right way, at the right time, or in the right place. For example, in his book, *Magical Medicine*, Wayland D. Hand points out that crossroads—or even just a fork in the road—have traditionally been considered magical places. Spirits and supernatural creatures are believed to gather there, and it is there that sick people are thought to be healed.

Don't Look Back

The taboo against looking backward is another important component of folk healing. For example, in North Carolina a folk cure for chicken pox dictates that the healer take the patient into a hog barn and then have him or her lie down and roll over three times. Next the patient must walk backward without turning around for 33 steps.

Among the Pennsylvania Dutch (farm people of German ancestry living in southeastern Pennsylvania), a person who wishes to get rid of a side ache, or "side stitch," must pick up a stone, spit on it, and throw it over his or her head without looking behind to see where the stone lands.

Numbers and Healing

Numbers also play an important role in folk medicine. Apparently, the number 3 has great religious significance, reflecting Christianity's Trinity of the Father, the Son, and the Holy Spirit. In North Carolina, for example, a folk cure for malaria directs the patient to "put a toad under a pot and walk around the pot three times," according to volume 6 of the *Frank C. Brown Collection of North Carolina Folklore.*

A precaution against backache documented by Brown advises that each spring, the first time an individual hears a dove's call, he or she should lie down and roll over on the ground three times.

Passing Through

Among the most primitive and long-lived folk remedies found through-out the world was the custom of pulling—or passing—patients through holes in trees, large stones, or other openings in natural or artificial objects. Although apparently rare compared to other forms of folk healing, the custom is rich in tradition.

In America, patients were most commonly made to crawl under the bellies of animals (usually donkeys); in some cases they were passed under table legs or through the rungs of ladders or other human-made objects, according to accounts documented in *Magical Medicine.*

In Vermont and New Hampshire, small children suffering from *hernias* (a protrusion of part of the intestine through the abdominal wall) were drawn through a split in a small tree, after which the halves of the tree were brought together again. The custom was based on the belief that if the tree healed properly so would the child's rupture. A similar folk cure for hernia was known in France at least as early as the 17th century.

Crawling or being pulled through briars and brambles is also common in folklore of various countries. It was a traditional cure for

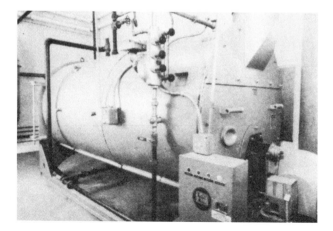

This "low temperature reflux high vacuum condenser" combines modern technology with ancient herbalism. The device is designed to remove and con-centrate active herbal ingredients.

whooping cough in Maryland, and in Europe the custom was used to treat children who were slow learners or to cure boils and other skin disorders. In England, this was considered a cure for *rheumatism* (joint pain), and the "remedy" was later transplanted to Texas.

BORN HEALERS

A circumstance of birth—being the seventh son of a father who was himself a seventh son—assumes an important role in folk medicine. The book *Magical Medicine* reports that in the Ozarks (rugged mountain country in the south-central United States, which includes parts of Missouri, Arkansas, Illinois, and Kansas), such a child is believed to be "endowed with healing powers which cannot be denied." When grown, that person is often referred to as Doc or Doctor.

A common belief in Europe, although less known in the United States, is that a child born with a *caul* (a portion of the membrane that surrounds the fetus before birth) covering his or her head is endowed with healing power. In Michigan, for example, believers claim that anyone born with a caul can stop another person's bleeding.

HEALING AND RELIGION

Religion and folk healing have a relationship dating back to ancient times, when people sought out their local holy man or woman to help with social, religious, family, and health problems.

Faith Healing

Today in rural America, *faith healers* routinely call upon the ill and frail to come to them and be treated by "healing hands." The laying on of hands, an ancient tradition adopted by Christianity, has thus made the long journey through the ages from the Old World to the New World.

Among some groups, such as the Louisiana Cajuns (descendants of immigrants from the French colony of Acadia), the tradition is passed on through the generations. Cajun healers, or *traiteurs*, do not usually

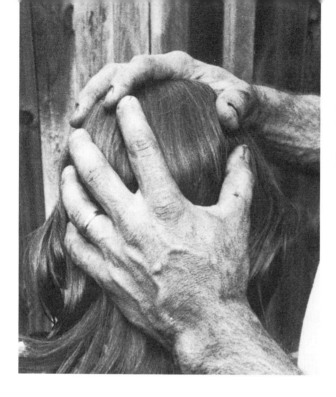

Healing through the laying on of hands is an ancient religious tradition that is still routinely practiced by faith healers.

claim the power to cure illnesses such as cancer and appendicitis. They do, however, use prayers, herbs, and touch to treat a variety of chronic problems including warts, *shingles* (a form of herpes), rashes, and lower back pain.

Some folk healers believe their power lies in the transfer of "good energies" into a patient and the simultaneous removal of "bad energies." This is somewhat similar to the Chinese folk medicine concept of reestablishing a proper balance of qi, the cosmic force flowing through the body that was discussed in Chapter 2.

Indeed, faith healing has found a place even in modern urban medical centers. Some hospitals in the New York City area, for example, are permitted to use faith healers to help win the confidence of mentally ill patients who are distrustful of modern psychiatric care, according to an article in *New York Newsday* (April 6, 1991).

Christian Science Healing

The belief in miraculous healing through religion exists today in many forms, but perhaps none so widely known as Christian Science.

Founded by Mary Baker Eddy in 1879, the religion's teachings are contained in her book *Science and Health with Key to the Scriptures.*

Eddy's Christian Science evolved during a period of deep introspection in her life following a series of personal misfortunes and ill health. Grappling with the question of God's responsibility for human suffering, she began to study the biblical stories of the healing powers of Jesus. Moreover, during this time she is believed to have recovered from a serious accident. Together, these events led her to found, with a group of followers, the Church of Christ, Scientist, for the purpose of reviving "primitive Christianity and its lost element of healing."

The church Eddy created emphasizes healing through prayer as part of a person's overall redemption from sin. Nevertheless, it also encourages its members to obey public health laws, and Christian Scientists regularly seek the services of physicians for setting bones or delivering babies. In recent years, however, Christian Science has come under increasing legal scrutiny following accounts of parents who have unsuccessfully used its spiritual healing practices to save their fatally ill children.

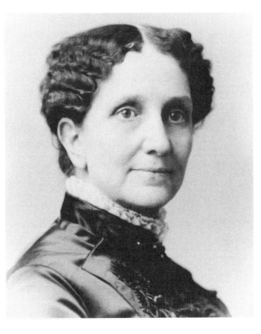

Mary Baker Eddy, founder of the Church of Christ, Scientist, espoused the power of healing through prayer.

A MODERN-DAY EXORCISM

A very dramatic incidence of religion-based healing, this time by the Roman Catholic church, also attracted attention not long ago. Audiences around the United States were captivated by a segment of the television show "20/20," which broadcast an exorcism performed on a 16-year-old girl. The subject, identified only as Gina, appeared to be suffering from mental illness but had not responded to standard treatment. The church, which today performs exorcisms on an infrequent basis, eventually ruled that the young woman was a victim of demonic possession, and a rite to dispel these demons was carried out in October 1990 (a videotape of the event was broadcast in April 1991).

The Roman Catholic church carefully regulates these rituals through its *canon* (laws). An exorcism is performed by a priest, who

The ancient ritual of exorcism, though not commonly practiced in modern times, is still conducted on occasion by the Roman Catholic church.

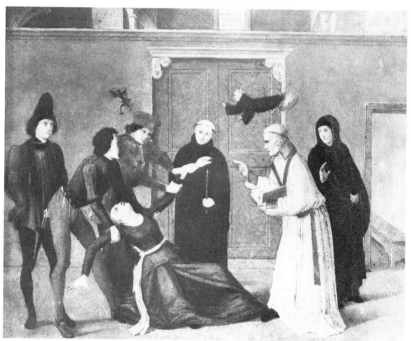

can conduct the ceremony only with a bishop's consent. A careful investigation must be made prior to the ritual to determine whether an individual is, in the church's opinion, a true victim of possession.

HEALING BASED ON NUTRITION

Health foods—those foods claimed to improve health and prevent or even cure disease—have a history dating back to ancient times. Certain foods have always been thought to have superior properties. Native Americans and Inuit, for example, believed that the brains, eyes, and glands of birds and other animals were particularly good for health and vitality.

Early concepts of health food may have developed in primitive agricultural communities with little or no access to certain foods containing essential minerals, vitamins, or amino acids according to the *Foods and Nutrition Encyclopedia* (first edition, 1983). The encyclopedia suggests that the sudden availability of a missing food, which would subsequently cure a severe nutritional deficiency, probably led to the belief in some communities that this food has special curative properties.

The promotion of healthy foods by early advocates such as John Harvey Kellogg (1852–1943) helped lead to today's multi-billion-dollar health food industry. Kellogg ran a health clinic where clients could enjoy a regimen of fresh air, exercise, and a special vegetarian diet. His brother, W. K. Kellogg (1860–1951), who was working with John to develop health foods for the clinic menu, invented Kellogg's Corn Flakes and went on to become rich in the breakfast cereal market.

Whether they are used to avoid the pesticides and preservatives in many other foods or to help gain athletic prowess, various products have been touted by the health food industry as having special curative or health-preserving properties. The true value of some of these choices varies, however.

For example, acidophilus milk—milk to which *Lactobacillus acidophilus* bacteria has been added—does appear to be beneficial. It has been found to help discourage harmful microorganisms from growing inside the intestines.

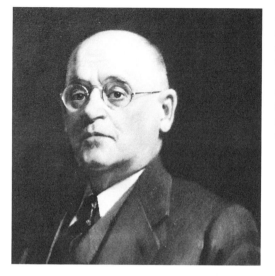

In an effort to create new foods for his brother John's health clinic, W. K. Kellogg invented Kellogg's Corn Flakes and went on to become wealthy in the breakfast cereal industry.

On the other hand, alfalfa flour, which is an excellent source of protein, calcium, and trace minerals, as well as vitamins E and K, is used by some health food enthusiasts for the treatment of diabetes. There is no evidence, however, that alfalfa is effective against this disease. In addition, some health food promoters claim that *lecithin*, a fatty substance contained in egg yolks and certain oils, such as soybean oil, will prevent or cure a variety of ills including arthritis, heart disease, and skin disorders. But again, there is no scientific proof of these assertions.

Other unproven claims would have consumers believe that flower pollen is good for general health and vitality, that *royal jelly* (the substance that worker bees feed to queen bees) rejuvenates sexuality, and that *blackstrap molasses* (molasses residue from sugar refining) can cure anemia and rheumatism.

NATUROPATHS: CHARLATANS OR TRUE HEALERS?

Perhaps the most organized and well-trained practitioners of unconventional medicine in the United States are the *naturopathic* doctors, or *naturopaths*. These healers use natural agents to combat disease and to restore or maintain a patient's health. Their treatment strategies include massage and other physical therapies, health counseling, herbal medicine, and attention to good nutrition.

An additional form of treatment, *hydrotherapy* (water therapy), is practiced in order to apply or reduce heat in various parts of the body. For example, wet heat helps relieve pain and improves the circulation of blood. Wet cold decreases body temperature and reduces blood flow, thus reducing swelling.

Naturopathic Training

Unlike most other forms of nonconventional healing, naturopathy is taught in a number of four-year graduate colleges specifically dedicated to the field and degrees in the subject are regularly awarded. The naturopathic student spends the first two years of his or her training studying basic medical science and much of the last two years in a naturopathic clinic learning to treat patients.

The Naturopathic Controversy

Among the many disputes between medical doctors and naturopaths is that of the role of nutrition in health. Naturopaths claim that nutritional remedies can bolster the immune system. However, William Bennett, M.D., editor of the *Harvard Medical School Health Letter,* referred to that assertion as "simply not supportable," according to the *Medical Tribune* (October 13, 1988).

Naturopaths also assert that herbal remedies can be safer than conventional drugs. According to these practitioners, when modern science synthesizes the active ingredients found in plants, the resulting medicine may be more toxic than it would be in its natural, unconcentrated state. Dr. Bennett again disputes this, characterizing the claim as nothing more than invalid "19th-century romantic philosophy."

Thus there is a complex debate between naturopaths and the medical profession. Naturopaths can present patients who testify to the success of this form of treatment, and in response, medical doctors claim that these healers simply present the apparent successes without bringing their failures forward as well.

Nevertheless, naturopathic medicine appears to be holding its own. Naturopathic colleges are producing dozens of graduates each year in the United States, and by the early 1990s, seven states were licensing these alternative doctors. In addition, although many physicians discount naturopathic claims concerning the superiority of herbal remedies, an herbalist from a naturopathic college was invited to speak at a student-sponsored lecture in 1987 at the Yale University School of Medicine.

FALSE CURES AND FALSE HOPE

Of all the diseases that plague humans, perhaps few are more terrifying to the general public than cancer is. Not suprisingly, then, there have been many different folk remedies touted as cures for various forms of this disease over the years.

Recently, one such "cure" was the oral administration of *laetrile*—a natural substance obtained from apricot pits. In the body, laetrile breaks down into several products, including *cyanide*, a powerful poison. A 1982 report in the *New England Journal of Medicine*, however, stated that a comprehensive study of laetrile found no basis for the claim that it could cure cancer.

In 1985, another study in the journal reported that large doses of vitamin C, also a supposed remedy for cancer, were useless as well (although scientific evidence does indicate that appropriate amounts of vitamin C may diminish the chance of getting certain types of cancer).

These few examples of cancer-cure quackery illustrate the more insidious side of folk medicine. Although there is a real basis for some of the remedies discussed in this book, the oftentimes desperate search for cures by those who either have little access to modern medical treatment or who prefer to supplement or substitute such care with folk remedies can lead to a fatal outcome.

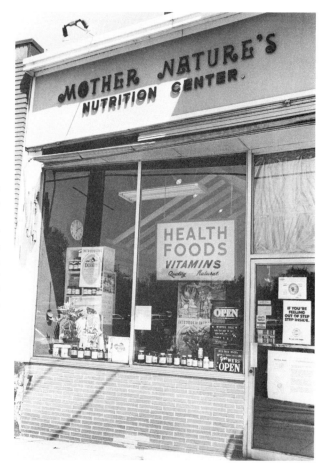

Health foods have evolved into a multi-billion-dollar industry, but consumers must be cautious. Although many foods are beneficial, the preventive or curative qualities of some have not been proved.

Such frantic searches continue to this day. A case in point is the growing number of people suffering from *acquired immune deficiency syndrome* (AIDS), which strips people of their immune defenses. Faced with almost certain, slow death, many AIDS patients will grasp at any potential remedy. Typhus vaccine, tea made from Brazilian tree bark, huge doses of antibiotics—even pond scum and a bed of electrically charged coils—have all been touted as cures for the deadly disease.

Unfortunately, it can be difficult to stop quack cures from being marketed to the public. Not only do laws on health fraud vary from state to state, but government agencies meant to protect consumers often do not have the funding needed to do an effective job. The FDA and other federal, state, and local government agencies are trying to educate the public on the subject of health fraud through a variety of means, including radio and television interviews, seminars, and presentations to consumer groups.

CONCLUSION

The lure of folk medicine is strong—and will probably remain so into the foreseeable future—because this type of treatment responds to the needs of those people who are either without access to sophisticated medical care or who are simply without hope. Folk medicine also appeals to those who wish to avoid the complex world of chemicals and technology and the sometimes impersonal physicians who practice modern medicine. These individuals prefer to seek help from the simple, people-oriented remedies that make up the wide variety of folk cures found throughout the world.

More than simply providing an alternative to Western health care, however, folk medicine also serves as a potential source of valuable "new" remedies, plant-based cures culled from herbal medications that have been successfully utilized for centuries. The ancient healing arts, then, promise to provide a legacy that stretches far into the future.

APPENDIX:
FOR MORE INFORMATION

The following is a list of organizations that can provide further information about folk medicine and related topics.

GENERAL INFORMATION

American Association for World Health
2021 L Street NW, Suite 250
Washington, DC 20036
(202) 265-0286

National Healthcare Antifraud
    Association
1255 23rd Street NW
Washington, DC 20037
(202) 659-5955

ACUPUNCTURE

Acupuncture Foundation of Canada
57 Simcoe Street South, Suite 2M
Oshawa, Ontario L1H 7N1
Canada
(416) 723-8970

Acupuncture Research Institute
313 West Andrix Street
Monterey Park, CA 91754
(213) 722-7353

International College of Acupunture and
    Electro-Therapeutics
(212) 781-6262

Traditional Acupuncture Institute
American City Building, Suite 100
Columbia, MD 21044
(301) 997-4888

AIDS

Federal Center for AIDS
301 Elgin Street, 2nd floor
Ottawa, Ontario K1A 0L2
Canada
Attn: Joel Finley
(613) 954-8500

People with AIDS Coalition
263A West 19th Street, #125
New York, NY 10011
(212) 532-0568

CANCER

American Cancer Society
1599 Clifton Road NE
Atlanta, GA 30329
1-800-ACS-2345

Memorial Sloan-Kettering Cancer
    Center
1275 York Avenue

New York, NY 10021
(212) 639-2000

HERBAL MEDICINE

American Herb Association
P.O. Box 1673
Nevada City, CA 95959

Herb Research Foundation
1007 Pearl Street, Suite 200
Boulder, CO 80302
(303) 449-2265

MASSAGE

American Massage Therapy
  Association
1130 West North Shore Avenue
Chicago, IL 60626-4670
(312) 761-2682

TAOISM

Daoist Sanctuary
P.O. Box 27806
Tempe, AZ 85285
(602) 839-5832

FURTHER READING

GENERAL INFORMATION

Atkinson, Donald T. *Magic, Myth and Medicine*. Salem, NH: Ayer, 1972.

Boulas, Loutfy. *Medicinal Plants of North Africa*. Algonac, MI: Reference, 1983.

Brown, Frank C. *The Frank C. Brown Collection of North Carolina Folklore, 7 vols.* Edited by Newman I. White. Durham, NC: Duke University Press, 1952–64.

Davis, Wade. *Passage of Darkness: The Ethnobiology of the Haitian Zombie*. Chapel Hill: University of North Carolina Press, 1988.

———. *The Serpent and the Rainbow: A Harvard Scientist Uncovers the Startling Truth About the Secret World of Voodoo and Zombies*. New York: Warner Books, 1987.

DeVries, Jan. *Traditional Home and Herbal Remedies*. New York: State Mutual Books, 1987.

Eddy, Mary Baker. *Science and Health with Key to the Scriptures*. Boston: First Church, 1875.

Gerrick, David J., and Doreen Dietsche. *Old Time Cures—Farmers Folklore*. Lorain, OH: Dayton Laboratories, 1980.

Hammerschlag, Carl A. *The Dancing Healers—A Doctor's Journey of Healing with Native Americans*. New York: HarperCollins, 1988.

Hand, Wayland D. *Magical Medicine: The Folkloric Component of Folk Medicine in the Folk Belief, Custom, and Ritual of the Peoples of Europe and America.* Berkeley: University of California Press, 1980.

Imperato, Pascal James. *African Folk Medicine: Practices and Beliefs of the Bambara and Other Peoples.* Parkton, MD: York Press, 1977.

Jarvis, D. C. *Folk Medicine.* New York: Fawcett Books, 1985.

Laguerre, Michael S. *Afro-Caribbean Folk Medicine: The Reproduction and Practice of Healing.* Granby, MA: Bergin & Garvey, 1987.

Lambo, J. O. *Catalogue of African Herbs.* Buffalo: Trado-Medic, N. d.

Leung, Albert Y. *Chinese Herbal Remedies.* New York: Universe, 1984.

McKenzie, Dan. *The Infancy of Medicine: Influence of Folklore upon Scientific Medicine.* New York: Gordon, 1977.

Meyer, Clarence. *American Folk Medicine.* Glenwood, IL: Meyerbooks, 1985.

Rinzier, Carol A. *The Dictionary of Medical Folklore.* New York: Ballantine, N. d.

Scarborough, John, ed. *Folklore and Folk Medicines.* Madison, WI: American Institute of the History of Pharmacy, 1987.

Singer, Phillip, ed. *Traditional Healing: New Science or New Colonialism? Essays in Critique of Medical Anthropology.* Buffalo: Trado-Medic, 1977.

Steiner, Richard P., ed. *Folk Medicine: The Art and the Science.* Washington, DC: American Chemical Society, 1985.

Touchstone, Samuel J. *Herbal Folk Medicine of Louisiana and Adjacent States.* Honolulu: Folk-Life, 1983.

AYURVEDIC MEDICINE

Dash, Bhagavan D. *Ayurvedic Cures for Common Diseases.* Pomona, CA: Auromere, 1986.

Dash, Vaidya B. *Fundamentals of Ayurvedic Medicine.* Flushing, NY: Asia Book Corp., 1980.

Gupta, Nagendranath S. *The Ayurvedic System of Medicine.* New York: Apt Books, 1975.

Lad, Vasant. *Ayurveda, the Science of Self-healing: A Practical Guide.* Wilmot, WI: Lotus Light, 1984.

Sharma, Shir. *The System of Ayurveda.* New York: Apt Books, 1983.

Tillotson, Alan K., et al. *The Handbook of Ayurvedic Medicine.* Virginia Beach: Grunwald & Radcliff, 1986.

SHAMANISM

Achterberg, Jeanne. *Imagery in Healing: Shamanism and Modern Medicine.* Boston: Shambhala, 1985.

Dioszegi, V., and M. Hoppal. *Shamanism in Siberia.* New York: State Mutual Books, 1978.

Grim, John. *Reflections on Shamanism: The Tribal Healer and the Technological Trance.* Chambersburg, PA: Anima, 1981.

Harner, Michael J., ed. *Hallucinogens and Shamanism.* New York: Oxford University Press, 1973.

Maddox, J. L. *The Medicine Man: A Sociological Study of the Character and Evolution of Shamanism.* New York: Gordon, 1977.

T'AI CHI

Chen, Y. K. *T'ai-Chi-Ch'uan: Its Effects and Practical Applications*. North Hollywood, CA: Newcastle, 1979.

Cheng, Man-Ch'ing, and Robert W. Smith. *T'ai Chi the Supreme Ultimate Exercise for Health, Sport, and Self-defense*. Rutland, VT: Tuttle, 1967.

Kauz, Herman. *T'ai Chi Handbook: Exercise, Meditation, Self-defense*. New York: Doubleday, 1974.

Lee, Douglas. *T'ai Chi Ch'uan the Philosophy of Yin and Yang and Its Applications*. Edited by Charles Lucas. Burbank: Ohara, 1976.

Stone, Justin F. *T'ai Chi Chih! Joy Thru Movement*. Rolling Hills Estates, CA: Satori Resources, 1986.

TAOISM

Blofeld, John. *Taoism: The Road to Immortality*. Boston: Shambhala, 1979.

Chang Po-tuan, and Liu I-Ming. *The Inner Teachings of Taoism*. Translated by Thomas Cleary. Boston: Shambhala, 1986.

Cooper, J. C. *Taoism: The Way of the Mystic*. York Beach, ME: Samuel Weiser, 1973.

Liu I-Ming. *Awakening to the Tao*. Edited by Kendra Crossen. Translated by Thomas Cleary. Boston: Shambhala, 1988.

Rawson, Philip, and Laszlo Legeza. *Tao: The Chinese Philosophy of Time and Change*. New York: Thames Hudson, 1984.

GLOSSARY

AIDS acquired immune deficiency syndrome; an acquired defect in the immune system; the final stage of the disease caused by the human immunodeficiency virus (HIV); spread by the blood, by sexual contact, through nutritive fluids passed from a mother to her fetus, or through breast milk; leaves victims vulnerable to certain, often fatal, infections and cancers

allicin extract of garlic; used as a Chinese home remedy to treat bacterial and fungal infections

amulet a charm worn to protect the wearer against evil forces, such as witchcraft or sorcery, or to aid him or her in such endeavors as love or war

anabolic steroids drugs, similar to the male hormone testosterone, that can increase muscle mass

antibiotic a substance that can destroy or inhibit the growth of microorganisms; used to treat infectious diseases

ayahuasca yage; a powerful hallucinogenic beverage prepared from the stem bark of the *Banisteriopsis caapi* vine

Ayurveda an ancient medical system practiced in India and parts of northern Asia; ayurvedic treatments include prescribed diets and herbal remedies

bhasmas ayurvedic medicines derived from metals and marine and animal products

bhutas according to the ayurvedic system, the five primary elements—e arth, water, light, air, and ether—that compose the human body and the universe

bokor a Haitian Voodoo sorcerer

caul a membrane that sometimes covers a child's head at birth

Church of Christ, Scientist Christian Science; a religion, founded by Mary Baker Eddy in 1879, that emphasizes healing of disease by mental and spiritual means

cupping as performed by African folk healers, supposedly involves sucking the "material" in a wound out through a cow horn

curare an extract of the *Strychnos toxifera* vine, used as a muscle relaxant

curative object an object worn by patients of African folk healers as an assurance that they will be cured

dhanvantari ghrita a substance made from plant juices and butter used as an ayurvedic treatment for diabetes

dhatus the seven tissues of ayurvedic medicine: plasma, blood, muscle, fat, bone, bone marrow, and semen

diviner a religious-medical specialist who is able to diagnose diseases and determine their causes through contact with spirits; supposedly possesses the ability to break spells cast by witch doctors

doshas the three substances—air, fire, and water—that, according to the teachings of ayurvedic medicine, determine human physical attributes

empirical knowledge knowledge gained by observation and experience

endorphins a group of pain-relieving proteins found in the brain

ethnobotanists scientists who study the plant lore of a people or race

formulary a manual containing lists of medicinal substances and formulas

ginkgolide B a substance derived from an extract of the ginkgo plant—an herb used in Chinese medicine for thousands of years—that has been found to be effective in treating asthma and allergic inflammations

ginseng a perennial plant of the genus *Panax*; the plant's thick, often fork-shaped root is used in Chinese folk medicine

healing cults groups that believe in the ability of spirits, saints, or specific human beings to heal others

herbalism the science of healing through the use of herbs

houngan the male leader of a Voodoo cult

hydrotherapy water therapy; the use of water to apply or reduce heat in the body

laetrile a drug derived from apricot pits that has been used unsuccessfully in cancer treatment

licorice the name applied to about a dozen plant species of the genus *Glycyrrhiza*, a member of the pea family; one species, *Glycyrrhiza glabra*, supplies a root used extensively in Chinese folk medicine to relieve sore throats, coughs, heart palpitations, stomachaches, ulcers, and sores

loa Voodoo gods that act as guardian angels

lwallichii a plant used in Japan and China to increase circulation through clogged blood vessels; has also been found to prevent blindness caused by the degeneration of the optic nerve and the retina

mahuang a Chinese medicinal herb that contains ephedrine, a substance used to relieve asthma, hay fever, and nasal congestion and to raise blood pressure

malas a term used in ayurvedic medicine to describe the body's waste products

mambo the female leader of a Voodoo cult

massage manipulating, kneading, or applying pressure to the body to relieve pain and tension

medicine man the priestly healer or sorcerer in American Indian tribes

narcotic a drug that dulls the senses, relieves pain, and induces sleep

naturopath a healer who treats disease through the use of natural agents instead of drugs

oricha/santo god/saint; the deity worshipped by followers of Santeria

peyote a drug that produces intoxication and feelings of ecstasy; used by North American Indians to enable them to converse with God and the spirits

placebo effect an improvement in a patient's condition resulting from his or her belief that the treatment administered is effective, rather than from the true value of the treatment itself

psychedelic capable of producing abnormal effects such as hallucinations

qi the force that governs changes in the human body, according to Chinese folk medicine

reserpine a drug derived from the snakeroot plant that is used to treat high blood pressure and mental disorders

Santería an Afro-Cuban religion containing elements of magic and Catholicism; Santerían belief holds that the religion's various gods control disease and that sickness can be cured by appeasing these dieties

shaman in Siberian and other north Asian cultures, a priest who cures the sick with the help of guardian spirits and who escorts the souls of the dead to the afterlife

snake cult a secret society whose members claim to be able to make their clients immune to snake bites

sorcerers in Africa, men who use "bad magic" to bring harm to their victims

sweat-emetic a Navajo ceremony performed to cure patients of their ailments by forcing them to vomit from the ingestion of an emetic and then to sweat from the heat of a fire

T'ai chi an ancient Chinese discipline consisting of a series of slow body movements thought by practitioners to balance yin/yang and promote good health

talisman an object engraved with a sign or character that acts as a charm to fend off evil and attract good fortune

Tao a Chinese philosophy that examines the way all things in nature change

traiteur a Louisiana Cajun healer who uses prayers, herbs, and touch to treat chronic illnesses

vaidya a skilled practitioner of ayurvedic medicine

Voodoo a cult that combines Western religion, Haitian and African beliefs, and drug use; initiates must undergo ceremonies that involve sacrifices to spirits, and followers direct their rituals toward guardian angels called loa

witch doctor an evil diviner who casts spells to bring harm to his clients' enemies

witch a woman, born with sinister powers, who uses her abilities to bring harm to her enemies

yin/yang the two opposite forces of nature; yin is the hard, feminine side, representing darkness and death; yang is the soft, masculine, side, representing light and life

yoga a system of exercises designed to attain physical or mental control and well-being; introduced in ancient India and practiced by Hindu priests as a means to clear the mind for prayer

zombie a person who is thought to have died and who is then reanimated

INDEX

PICTURE CREDITS

Marc Kusinitz is a science writer for the Public Affairs Department at the University of Maine in Orono. He holds an M.S. in environmental health sciences from the University of Rhode Island and a Ph.D. in biology from New York University. Previously, Dr. Kusinitz was a science journalist whose work appeared in the *San Jose Mercury News*, *Technology Review*, and the *New York Times*, among other publications. He is a past news editor of the *New York State Journal of Medicine* and served as both editor and writer for *New Medical Science*, a monthly publication for physicians.

Dale C. Garell, M.D., is medical director of California Children Services, Department of Health Services, County of Los Angeles. He is also associate dean for curriculum at the University of Southern California School of Medicine and clinical professor in the Department of Pediatrics & Family Medicine at the University of Southern California School of Medicine. From 1963 to 1974, he was medical director of the Division of Adolescent Medicine at Children's Hospital in Los Angeles. Dr. Garell has served as president of the Society for Adolescent Medicine, chairman of the youth committee of the American Academy of Pediatrics, and as a forum member of the White House Conference on Children (1970) and White House Conference on Youth (1971). He has also been a member of the editorial board of the *American Journal of Diseases of Children*.

C. Everett Koop, M.D., Sc.D., is former Surgeon General, deputy assistant secretary for health, and director of the Office of International Health of the U.S. Public Health Service. A pediatric surgeon with an international reputation, he was previously surgeon-in-chief of Children's Hospital of Philadelphia and professor of pediatric surgery and pediatrics at the University of Pennsylvania. Dr. Koop is the author of more than 175 articles and books on the practice of medicine. He has served as surgery editor of the *Journal of Clinical Pediatrics* and editor-in-chief of the *Journal of Pediatric Surgery*. Dr. Koop has received nine honorary degrees and numerous other awards, including the Denis Brown Gold Medal of the British Association of Paediatric Surgeons, the William E. Ladd Gold Medal of the American Academy of Pediatrics, and the Copernicus Medal of the Surgical Society of Poland. He is a chevalier of the French Legion of Honor and a member of the Royal College of Surgeons, London.